T0282632

CAMBRIDGE LIBRARY COLLECTION

Books of enduring scholarly value

History of Medicine

It is sobering to realise that as recently as the year in which On the Origin of Species was published, learned opinion was that diseases such as typhus and cholera were spread by a 'miasma', and suggestions that doctors should wash their hands before examining patients were greeted with mockery by the profession. The Cambridge Library Collection reissues milestone publications in the history of Western medicine as well as studies of other medical traditions. Its coverage ranges from Galen on anatomical procedures to Florence Nightingale's common-sense advice to nurses, and includes early research into genetics and mental health, colonial reports on tropical diseases, documents on public health and military medicine, and publications on spa culture and medicinal plants.

Introductory Notes on Lying-In Institutions

The greatest postnatal killer of the nineteenth century was puerperal fever. A vicious and usually fatal form of septicaemia, puerperal or childbed fever was known to occur in maternity hospitals far more frequently than at home births, and to spread faster in crowded wards than in those with fewer patients. Its cause was unknown. In this precise statistical analysis of the facts, gathered from several sources across the major cities of Europe, Florence Nightingale (1820–1910) explores the mystery of puerperal fever and its possible causes. She stresses the necessity of good ventilation in hospitals, condemning those with overcrowded wards, and cites instances where the layout of wards has a noticeable correlation with the number of deaths. Published in 1871, just before Pasteur's work on germ theory proved that the problem could be all but eradicated if doctors washed their hands more rigorously, this work remains clear, scholarly and engaging.

Introductory Notes on Lying-In Institutions

*Together with a Proposal
for Organising an Institution
for Training Midwives
and Midwifery Nurses*

FLORENCE NIGHTINGALE

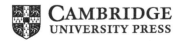
CAMBRIDGE
UNIVERSITY PRESS

CAMBRIDGE UNIVERSITY PRESS

Cambridge, New York, Melbourne, Madrid, Cape Town,
Singapore, São Paolo, Delhi, Mexico City

Published in the United States of America by Cambridge University Press, New York

www.cambridge.org
Information on this title: www.cambridge.org/9781108053198

© in this compilation Cambridge University Press 2012

This edition first published 1871
This digitally printed version 2012

ISBN 978-1-108-05319-8 Paperback

ON

LYING-IN INSTITUTIONS.

LONDON : PRINTED BY
SPOTTISWOODE AND CO., NEW-STREET SQUARE
AND PARLIAMENT STREET

INTRODUCTORY NOTES

ON

LYING-IN INSTITUTIONS.

TOGETHER WITH

A PROPOSAL FOR
ORGANISING AN INSTITUTION FOR TRAINING MIDWIVES
AND MIDWIFERY NURSES.

BY

FLORENCE NIGHTINGALE.

LONDON:

LONGMANS, GREEN, AND CO.

1871.

IF I may dedicate, without 'permission,' these small 'Notes' to the shade of Socrates' Mother, may I likewise, without presumption, call to my help the questioning shade of her Son, that I who write may have the spirit of questioning aright, and that those who read may learn not of me but of themselves?

And, further, has he not said: 'The midwives are respectable women, and have a character to lose'?

PREFACE.

In the year 1862 the Committee of the Nightingale Fund, with a view to extending the advantages of their Training Institution, entered into an arrangement with the authorities of St. John's House, under which wards were fitted up in the new part of King's College Hospital, opening out of the great staircase and shut up within their own doors, for the reception of Midwifery cases. The wards were under the charge of the (then) Lady Superintendent. Arrangements were made for medical attendance, a skilled midwife was engaged, a certain number of pupil nurses were admitted for training; and hopes were entertained that this new branch of our Training School would confer a great benefit on the poor, especially in country districts, where trained Midwifery nurses are needed.

Every precaution had apparently been taken to render the Midwifery Department perfectly safe; and it was not until the school had been upwards of five years in existence, that the attention of the Nightingale Committee was called to the fact that deaths from puerperal diseases had taken place in each of the preceding years.

During the period of nearly six years that the wards were in use, the records show that 780 women had been delivered in the institution, and that out of this number twenty-six * had died—a mortality of 33·3 per 1,000.

The most fatal year was 1867, in which year nine out of the twenty-six deaths took place. In the month of January a pregnant woman, who was under treatment for erysipelas in the hospital, was delivered in a general medical ward, No. 4, in the first-built wing of the hospital. A midwife was told off to attend her, who was not suffered to be near the midwifery wards for a considerable time. The erysipelas case died of puerperal fever; and this death was followed by a succession of puerperal deaths in the lying-in wards until November, when the wards were as soon as possible closed.

An analysis of the causes of death showed that, with the exception of one death from hæmorrhage, not a single death had taken place from accidents incidental to child-bearing during the whole six years. There were three deaths due to diseases not necessarily concomitants of this condition; while of the others, twenty-three in number, no fewer than seventeen were due to puerperal fever, three to puerperal peritonitis, two to pyæmia, and one to metritis.

---

* Exclusive of the case of a poor woman who was delivered in a cab, and died in the hospital of *post partum* hæmorrhage.

The following table gives the actual fates and dates :—

Midwifery Statistics, King's College Hospital.

Year	Total Deliveries	Date of Birth	Nature of Labour	Cause of Death	Date of Death	Deaths to Labours
				Fatal Cases		
1862	97	Nov. 6	Natural	Puerperal peritonitis	Nov. 25	⎫
		,, 30	Twins	{ Phthisis and puerperal fever }	Dec. 27	⎬ 1 in 32·3
		Dec. 10	Natural	Puerperal peritonitis	Dec. 20	⎭
1863	105	Jan. 10	{ Natural. Child still-born }	Puerperal fever	Jan. 16	⎬ 1 in 52·5
		April 29	Natural	Puerperal fever	May 20	
1864	141	Feb. 16	Natural	Puerperal fever	Feb. 25	
		April 14	Induced	Pyæmia	April 29	⎬ 1 in 47
		Dec. 1	Born in cab	Hæmorrhage	Dec. 7	
1865	163	Jan. 30	Natural	Embolism	Feb. 12	⎫
		Feb. 8	Natural	Puerperal fever	Feb. 18	
		June 24	Forceps	{ Puerperal metritis and pelvis cellulitis }	July 30	⎬ 1 in 32·6
		Oct. 20	Forceps	{ Laceration of perinæum, puerperal fever }	Nov. 3	
		Oct. 29	Natural	Puerperal fever	Nov. 9	⎭
1866	150	Jan. 10	Natural	Gastro-enteritis	Jan. 20	⎫
		Mar. 24	Natural	{ Retained placenta, puerperal fever }	April 10	
		Oct. 8	{ Placenta prævia. Turning }	Emphysema and bronchitis	Oct. 10	⎬ 1 in 30
		Nov. 10	Forceps	Peritonitis	Nov. 15	
		Dec. 4	Natural	Puerperal fever	Dec. 31	⎭
1867	125	Jan. 10	{ (Had erysipelas when admitted*) }	Puerperal fever	Jan. 30	⎫
		Feb. 7	Natural	{ Considerable hæmorrhage, puerperal fever }	Feb. 22	
		,, 8	Natural	Puerperal fever	Feb. 22	
		April 12	Turning	Puerperal fever	April 22	
		May 18	Natural	Pyæmia	May 27	⎬ 1 in 13·8
		June 4	Natural	Puerperal fever	June 19	
		July 26	Natural	Puerperal fever	Aug. 11	
		Nov. 5	{ Twins : 1st dead, 2nd by turning }	Puerperal fever	Nov. 10	
		,, 8	Forceps	{ Laceration of vagina, puerperal fever }	Nov. 14	⎭
Total	781	—	—	—	deaths : 27	1 in 28·9

* ' So was confined in No. 4 ward.'

Under these deplorable circumstances the closing of the wards was a matter of course ; and since that event we have been anxiously enquiring whether it would be justifiable to re-open our Midwifery Nursing School under other conditions.

This question is discussed in the following pages, from a basis of statistical facts supplied by the best authorities; and a few proposals have been added, with the view of turning to the best account our past experience, by extracting from it any leading principles which may present themselves for practical application in the future construction and management of Lying-in Institutions, and more especially in connection with means of training Midwifery nurses.

These Introductory Notes, collected and put together under circumstances of all but overwhelming business and illness, are now thrown out merely as a nucleus, in the hope that others will be kind enough to supplement, to add, and to alter; in fact, only as a hook with a modest little fish on it—a bait to catch other and finer fish.

The facts themselves, the nucleus, have been made as correct as it was possible, and as would have been done for a finished work. But the facts themselves are only put forth as feelers—feelers to feel my own way.

I need scarcely say either that these 'Notes' are not at all meant to discuss every point which presents itself in Midwifery statistics. On the contrary, they are, for the moment, purposely limited to the consideration of facts immediately relating to the present object.

Let me thank once more with true gratitude all those who have so kindly supplied me with help and information, some of whose names will appear in the following pages.

CONTENTS.

———◆◇◆———

CHAPTER II.

LIST OF PLANS.

NOTES

ON

LYING-IN INSTITUTIONS.

——•◦•——

THE FIRST STEP to be taken in the discussion is to enquire,
What is the real normal death-rate of lying-in women? And,
having ascertained this to the extent which existing data
may enable us to do, we must compare this death-rate with
the rates occurring in establishments into which parturition
cases are received in numbers. We have then to classify
the causes of death, so far as we can, from the data, with the
view of ascertaining whether any particular cause of death
predominates in lying-in institutions; and, if so, why so?
And finally, seeing that everybody must be born, that
every birth in civilised countries is as a rule attended by
somebody, and ought to be by a skilled attendant; since,
therefore, the attendance upon lying-in women is the widest
practice in the world, and these attendants should be trained;
we must decide the great question as to whether a training-
school for midwifery nurses can be safely conducted in any

building receiving a number of parturition cases, or whether such nurses must be only trained at the bedside in the patient's own home, with far more difficulty and far less chance of success.

MIDWIFERY STATISTICS.

It must be admitted, at the very outset of this enquiry, that midwifery statistics are in an unsatisfactory condition. To say the least of it, there has been as much discussion regarding mortality and its causes among lying-in women as there has been regarding the mortality due to hospitals. Yet there appears to have been no uniform system of record of deaths, or of the causes of death, in many institutions, and no common agreement as to the period after delivery within which deaths should be counted as due to the puerperal condition. Many of the most important institutions in Europe merely record the deaths occurring during the period women are in hospital, and they appear not unfrequently to do this without any reference to the causes. Similar defects are obvious enough in the records of home deliveries; and hence it follows that the mass of statistics which have been accumulated regarding home and hospital deliveries, admit of comparison only in one element, namely, the total deaths to total deliveries, and this only approximately.

Dr. Matthews Duncan, in his recent work on the 'Mortality of Childbed and Maternity Hospitals,' has dwelt forcibly on these defects in midwifery statistics, and has made out a strong case for improvement in records. But, as will be afterwards shown, with all their defects, midwifery statistics point to one truth ; namely, that there is a large amount of preventible mortality in midwifery practice, and that, as a general rule, the mortality is far, far greater in lying-in hospitals than among women lying-in at home.

There are several of what may be called secondary influences also, which must affect to a certain extent the results of comparison of death-rates among different groups of lying-in cases. Such are the ages of women, the number of the pregnancy, the duration of labour, and the like. It is impossible, in the present state of our information, to attribute to each, or all of these, their due influence ; neither, if we could do so, would it materially affect the general result just stated. But it is otherwise with another class of conditions, of which statistics take no cognizance. Such are the general sanitary state of hospitals, wards, houses, and rooms where deliveries take place ; the management adopted ; the classes of patients ; their state of health and stamina before delivery ; the time they are kept in midwifery wards before and after delivery. These elements are directly connected with the questions at issue, and yet our information regarding them is by no means so full as we could wish—indeed is almost nothing.

Our only resource at present is to deal with such statistical information as we possess, and to ascertain fairly what it tells us. This we shall now endeavour to do, beginning with an estimate of the normal mortality due to childbirth in various European countries.

NORMAL DEATH-RATE OF LYING-IN WOMEN IN ENGLAND.

In the Registrar-General's Thirtieth Annual Report, 1867, there is an instructive series of tables, giving approximately the present normal death-rate among lying-in women in England.

One of these tables (abstracted on Table I.) shows that, including deliveries in lying-in hospitals, there were in England, during the year 1867, 768,349 births, and that 3,933 women died in childbed. This gives an approximate total mortality of 5·1 per 1,000 from all causes.

TABLE I.—*Mortality after Childbirth in England*, 1867 (*Registrar-General's Thirtieth Annual Report*).

Total Births	Deaths from Accidents in Childbirth	Deaths from Puerperal Diseases	Deaths from Miasmatic Diseases	Deaths from Consumption and Chest Diseases	Deaths from all Other Causes	Total Deaths
768,349	2,346	1,066	137	230	154	3,933

The causes of mortality are also given in Table I. as follows :—

1. There were 2,346 deaths by accidents of childbirth (hæmorrhage, convulsions, exhaustion, mania, &c.).

2. There were 1,066 deaths due to puerperal diseases (puerperal fever, puerperal peritonitis, metritis, pyæmia, &c.).

3. Of the remaining 521 deaths, 137 were due to non-puerperal fevers and eruptive fevers; 230 were occasioned

by consumption and other chest diseases, and 154 by other causes.

4. By adding together deaths from puerperal diseases and those from fevers, we find that, out of a total mortality of 3,933, the deaths from diseases more or less connected with what is called 'blood-poisoning' amounted to 1,203, or rather more than 30 per cent. of the tot a mortality.

5. The mortality per 1,000 deliveries (or rather per 1,000 births) from each class of causes in England, in 1867, stands thus :—

Accidents of childbirth	.	.	.	. 3 per 1,000
Puerperal diseases .	.	.	.	. 1·4 „ „
Others, including non-puerperal fevers	.	.	·7 „ „
Total	.	.	.	. 5·1 „ „

The same Report gives the following puerperal death-rates for all England during 13 years, 1855 to 1867 (see Table II.).

Accidents of childbirth .	.	.	. 3·22 per 1,000
Puerperal diseases	.	.	. 1·61 „ „
Total, exclusive of other deaths .	.	4·83 „ „

An important element in the analysis of these death-rates is their relative prevalence in town and country. This is abstracted on Table II. from the Registrar-General's Report for a period of ten years, as follows :—

Deaths from Accidents of Childbirth and Puerperal Diseases.

England, 64 healthy districts, 312,402 deliveries . 4·3 per 1000
Ditto, 11 large towns, 1,402,304 deliveries . 4·9 „ „

In other words, out of every 5,000 deliveries in towns there are three more deaths from accidents of childbirth and puerperal diseases than occur among the same number of deliveries in healthy districts.

These facts, with a small deduction for the higher death-rates in lying-in hospitals, give the present mortality in English homes. They appear to show that puerperal women are subject to something of the same law of increase of death-rates in towns as other people, but part of the increase is no doubt due to the higher death-rates in delivery-wards in these towns. The facts also appear to indicate a probable reduction of death-rates among lying-in women in England, from the extension of public health improvements both in town and country.

TABLE II.—*Table Showing the Mortality per Thousand after Delivery from Puerperal Diseases and Accidents of Childbirth.*

Places	Mortality Per Thousand Deliveries		
	Puerperal Diseases	Accidents of Child-birth	Puerperal Diseases and Accidents of Childbirth
King's College lying-in ward, 5 years . .	29·4	0	29·4
12 Parisian Hospitals 1861 { . . .	—	—	75·2
1862 { . . .	—	—	56·7
1863 { . . .	—	—	60·6
Queen Charlotte's Lying-in Hospital, 40 years	14·3	5·3	19·6
27 London workhouses, in which both deliveries and deaths have taken place .	4·1	2 1	6·2
40 London workhouses, including those without deaths, 5 years	3·3	1·7	5·0
Liverpool Workhouse lying-in wards, 13 years	3·4	2·2	5·6
All England, 13 years . . .	1·61	3·22	4·83
Ditto, 64 healthy districts (312,402 deliveries), 10 years	—	—	4·3
Ditto, 11 large towns (1,402,304 deliveries), 10 years	—	—	4·9
8 military lying-in hospitals, 2 to 12 years .	3·9	3·4	7·3

NORMAL MORTALITY AMONG LYING-IN WOMEN IN DIFFERENT COUNTRIES.

The next step in the enquiry is to ascertain, so far as it may be possible to do so, what is the death-rate among lying-in women delivered at their own homes in different European countries. Besides the mortality statistics for healthy districts in England, already given, the only available data for this information are reports of public institutes having outdoor midwifery practice, and any records of private practice which may have been published. In adducing these data, however, it is necessary to do so with the reservation already made that their accuracy is only approximate.

The most extensive series of data of this class is given by Dr. Le Fort in his able treatise 'Des Maternites,' for a number of institutions in different European countries. The facts from Dr. Le Fort's book are abstracted on Table III., in which it is shown that out of 934,781 deliveries at home, in Edinburgh, London, Paris, Leipzic, Berlin, Munich, Greifswald, Stettin, and St. Petersburg, there were 4,405 deaths, equivalent to a mortality of 4·7 per 1,000. When compared with the Registrar-General's returns for town districts, this rate is apparently somewhat too low; it is only an approximation, but still sufficiently near the rate given by the Registrar-General to show that there is a true death-rate for home deliveries not far removed from the Registrar-General's figure.

TABLE III.—*Table Showing the Death-rate from all Causes amongst Women Delivered in their own Homes. (Abstracted from Dr. Le Fort's Tables.)*

Places	No. of Years of Observation	Deliveries	Deaths	Deaths per Thousand
Edinburgh . . .	1	5,186	28	5
London:				
Westminster General Dispensary . . .	11	7,717	17	2
Ditto Benevolent Institution .	7	4,761	8	1
Royal Maternity Charity .	5	17,242	53	3
London population . .	5	562,623	2,222	3·9
St. Thomas' Hospital . .	7	3,512	9	2·5
Guy's Hospital . .	8	11,928	36	3
Ditto	1	1,505	4	2
Ditto : . . .	1	1,702	3	1·7
Ditto : . .	1	1,576	11	6
Paris:				
12th Arrondissement . .	1	3,222	10	3
Bureau de Bienfaisance .	1	6,212	32	5
Ditto	1	6,422	39	6
City of Paris . . .	1	44,481	262	5
Ditto	1	42,796	226	5
Leipzig Polyclinique . .	11	1,203	13	10
Berlin „ . .	1	500	7	14
Munich „ . .	5	1,911	16	8
Greifswald „ . .	4	295	6	20
Stettin „ . .	17	375	0	0
St. Petersburg . . .	15	209,612	1,403	6·6
Total . . .	—	934,781	4,405	4·7

St. George's Hospital Statistics for ' the 6 years preceding 1870 show only one maternal death in every 305 cases ' in the Out-door Maternity Department.

From home records, it is hoped at some future time to give many more data of this kind, and to distinguish the causes of death: puerperal from non-puerperal mortality, as well as that caused by puerperal diseases from that caused by accidents of childbirth. At present the data for doing this are lamentably deficient, if not almost altogether wanting.

One good recorded fact will here be given. Among 1,929 mothers delivered at home by Guy's Hospital in 1869, 5 deaths only are recorded, and none from puerperal diseases; 2 were from heart disease, 2 from pneumonia, 1 from exhaustion.

OBJECTIONS TO THE DATA.

The value of the Registrar-General's results, and of those given by Le Fort, has been called in question by Dr. Duncan in his work already cited, partly on the authority of certain results of home practice, quoted from Dr. M'Clintock, who has collected the statistics of 16,774 deliveries exclusively from home practice. There were among these 45 deaths from accidents of labour, 52 deaths from puerperal diseases, and 34 deaths from non-puerperal diseases ; giving a total mortality of 131, or nearly 8 per 1,000. On considering these figures, the first impression they convey is not that either the Registrar-General or Le Fort is wrong. But it is a very painful impression of another kind altogether. One feels disposed to ask whether it can be true that, in the hands of educated accoucheurs, the inevitable fate of women undergoing, not a diseased, but an entirely natural condition, at home, is that one out of every 128 must die? If the facts are correct, then one cannot help feeling that they present a very strong *prima facie* case for enquiry, with the view of devising a remedy for such a state of things. It must be seen, however, that these statistics of home practice are as open to the charge of want of accuracy as those of the Registrar-General or Le Fort. The question can only be settled by enquiry, and by more carefully kept statistics of midwifery practice; but in the meantime here are a few facts, kindly placed at my disposal by Mr. Rigden, of Canterbury, which are by no means so hopeless as those given by Dr. Duncan.

' An analysis of 4,132 consecutive cases in midwifery occurring in private practice during a period of 30 years, particularly in reference to mortality. Eight mothers died: three from convulsions and coma; 4 from puerperal fever; and one from heart disease, about an hour after a comparatively easy labour.'

The report states 8, but after it was supplied another death took place, the day after delivery, making 9 in all. The cause of death is not given.

Mr. Rigden explains that these figures relate only to the first fortnight after delivery; but he states that if any other deaths had taken place within the month, he must have heard of them.

Assuming the Deliveries at 4,133 and the Deaths at 9, Mr. Rigden's facts show a total mortality of 2·17 per 1,000, of which less than 1 per 1,000 was due to puerperal fever.

ESTIMATED APPROXIMATE HOME DEATH-RATE.

In estimating the probable accuracy of statistical data in which there may be both excesses and deficiencies, sources of error are diminished by largeness in the numbers employed in striking averages. Bearing this in mind, and after considering the objections brought against the accuracy of the figures, there seems no reason for rejecting the Registrar-General's average total mortality among lying-in women in England of 5·1 per 1,000, as affording a sufficiently close approximation to the present real death-rate among lying-in women delivered at home, for all practical purposes of comparison with the death-rates in lying-in hospitals.

DEATH-RATES IN LYING-IN INSTITUTIONS.

We shall next show approximately what are the death-rates in establishments for lying-in women.

We will give an abstract of mortality statistics for a number of these institutions, the general results of which may be stated as follows :—

In eight military lying-in hospitals (Table IV.), in which 5575 deliveries took place, in periods of from 2 to 12 years, there were 50 deaths (excluding a death before admission) —a death-rate of 8·8 per 1,000.

TABLE IV.—Return of the Number of Admissions for Parturition, and Deaths occurring in the undermentioned Women's Hospitals (Military). (Supplied by the Director-General, Army Medical Department.)

Station	Period	No. of Deliveries	Puerperal Fever and Peritonitis, Pyæmia, Phlebitis, &c.	Scarlatina	Puerperal Convulsions	Hæmorrhage, Effects of	Ruptured Uterus	Syncope and Exhaustion	Premature Labour and Adherent Placenta	Craniotomy	Inversion of Uterus	Embolism	Metritis	Pneumonia and Bronchitis	Phthisis	Dropsy	Cause not recorded	Total Deaths
Devonport	April 1861 to Dec. 1869	158	—	—	1	—	—	—	—	—	—	—	—	—	—	—	—	1
Colchester	1865 to Oct. 1870	252	—	—	—	—	—	—	—	—	—	—	—	—	—	—	—	—
Portsmouth	1861 to Dec. 1869	302	2	—	1	—	—	—	—	1	—	—	—	—	—	—	—	4
Aldershot	1857 „	3,028	14	—	1	4	1	4	1	1	—	—	1*	2	1	—	1	31
Shorncliffe	Up to „ Dec. 1863	702	—	1	—	1	—	—	—	2	—	—	—	—	—	—	—	4
Chatham	Nov. 1863 „	342	—	2	—	—	—	—	—	—	1†	—	—	—	—	—	—	3
Woolwich	1868 and 1869	751	5‡	—	—	—	—	1	—	—	—	1	—	—	—	1	—	8
Curragh	·	40	—	—	—	—	—	—	—	—	—	—	—	—	—	—	—	—
Total	—	5,575	21	3	3	5	1	5	1	4	1	1	1	2	1	1	1	51

* Patient died 48 hours after delivery.   † Patient died on her way to the hospital : not included in the calculated rates.
‡ One case had gastric fever on admission, and in two cases puerperal peritonitis came on after instrumental delivery.

In Liverpool workhouse lying-in wards (Table V.), with an
approximate number of 6,396 deliveries in 13 years, there
were 58 deaths from all causes—a mortality of 9·06 per 1,000.

TABLE V.—*Statistics of Midwifery Wards in Liverpool Workhouse for Thirteen Years, 1858–70 inclusive. (Abstracted
from data supplied by Dr. Barnes, Liverpool.)*

Approximate Total Deliveries	Causes of Death																	Total Deaths
	Puerperal Peritonitis	Puerperal Fever	Metritis	Phlegmasia Dolens	Convulsions	Debility and Exhaustion	Obstructed Labour	Hæmorrhage	Rupture of Uterus	Typhus and Re-lapsing Fever	Measles	Pneumonia	Laryngitis	Phthisis	Heart Disease	Nephritic Disease and Dropsy	Jaundice and Bowel Disease	Not Stated (Inquest)	
6,396	16	4	1	1	5	5	1	2	1	2	1	3	1	4	5	3	2	1	58

And in 27 London workhouse infirmaries (Table VI.),
amongst which deaths took place, having 9,411 deliveries
in five years, there were 93 deaths from all causes. The
death-rate was 9·8 per 1,000.[1]

TABLE VI.—*Mortality after Childbirth in Five Years, up to the
end of 1865, in Forty London Workhouse Infirmaries in
which Deliveries took place. (Abstracted from Report on
Metropolitan Workhouses.)*

Deliveries	Deaths from Puerperal Diseases	Deaths from Accidents in Childbirth	Deaths from Miasmatic Diseases	Deaths from Consumption and Chest Diseases	Deaths from all Other Causes	Total Deaths
27 workhouses: 9,411	39	20	0	15	19	93
13 ,, 2,459	0	0	0	0	0	0

[1] In 1868, 69, 70, there were in Liverpool workhouse, 1,416 deliveries,
including 20 premature, and 6 deaths from all causes, of which 3 at least were
non-puerperal. The *total* death-rate was only 4·2 per 1,000. There were 13
London workhouses in which, in 5 years, 2,459 deliveries, but no deaths in
childbed, took place.

The City of London Lying-in Institution, during ten years, 1859–1868, had 4,966 deliveries, and 54 deaths—a rate of 10·9 per 1,000.

The British Lying-in Institution had 1,741 deliveries, and 25 deaths, in 11 years, 1858–1868, giving a death-rate of 14·3 per 1,000 (Table VIII.).

The mortality in Queen Charlotte's Lying-in Hospital: 9,626 deliveries, and 244 deaths, from 1828 to 1868 (Table VII.), was 25·3 per 1,000.

TABLE VII.—*Mortality in Queen Charlotte's Lying-in Hospital, 1828 to 1868.*

Deliveries	Deaths from Puerperal Diseases	Deaths from Accidents in Childbirth	Deaths from Miasmatic Diseases	Deaths from Consumption and Chest Diseases	Deaths from all Other Causes	Total Deaths
9,626	138	51	8	32	15	244

The Rotunda Hospital, Dublin, with 6,521 deliveries in the years 1857–1861, yielded 169 deaths—a death-rate of 26 per 1,000. But, if we take the years 1828–1861, with 63,621 deliveries, we find that the deaths were 924, and the death-rate only 14·5 per 1,000—the average annual number of deliveries being almost as many thousands as in Queen Charlotte's Hospital were hundreds.

TABLE VIII.—*Mortality per Thousand from all Causes after Delivery.* (*Abstracted from Official Reports and Returns.*)

Places	Deliveries	Deaths	Deaths per Thousand Deliveries
12 Parisian hospitals { 1861	7,309	—	95·1
1862	7,027	—	69·7
1863	7,289	—	70·3
King's College Hospital, 1862-7 . .	780*	26	33·3
Rotunda Hospital, Dublin, 1857-61 .	6,521	169	26·0
Queen Charlotte's Lying-in Hospital, 1828-68	9,626	244	25·3
British Lying-in Institution, 11 years, 1858 -68	1,741	25	14·3
City of London Lying-in Hospital, 1859-68	4,966	54	10·9
8 military lying-in hospitals, 2 to 12 years .	5,575	50	8·8
Liverpool Workhouse Lying-in Wards, 13 years, 1858-70	6,396	58	9·06
40 London workhouse infirmaries, 5 years .	11,870	93	7·8
1 military lying-in hospital (a wooden hut) 1865-70	252	0	0
All England, 1867	768,349	3,933	5·1

* Exclusive of a fatal case delivered in a cab.

The lying-in wards of King's College Hospital, years 1862-1867 (Table IX.), gave 27 deaths—a death-rate of 33·3 per 1,000 on 780 deliveries.

TABLE IX.—*Mortality after Childbirth in Lying-in Ward, King's College Hospital,* 1862 to 1867.

Deliveries	Deaths from Puerperal Diseases	Deaths from Accidents in Childbirth	Deaths from Miasmatic Diseases	Deaths from Consumption and Chest Diseases	Deaths from all Other Causes	Total Deaths
781*	23	1*	0	1	2	27

* One delivery took place in a cab, and the woman died in hospital.

Lamentable as are these death-rates in many British institutions, they are small in comparison with those which have ruled in many foreign hospitals.

Table X. contains an abstract from Dr. Le Fort's work of the statistics of 58 lying-in institutions in nearly every country of Europe, and extending in many cases over a considerable number of years. There is only one hospital (at Bourg) in which there was no death in 4 years, out of 461 deliveries.

There is one hospital (at Troyes), with a death-rate of 4 per 1,000 on 460 deliveries in 4 years.

There are two instances of death-rates of 7 per 1,000. There is one of 9, and there are two of 10 per 1,000.

In every other case the death-rates have exceeded these amounts, rising higher and higher in different institutions, until they culminate in a death-rate of no less than 140 per 1,000, at Strasburg, on a four years' average among 556 deliveries. Le Fort's data show a striking variation in the death-rates of the same hospitals in different years, as will presently be seen to be the case in hospitals in this country. There are instances in these foreign hospitals of the death rates varying from 4 to 7-fold in different groups of years in the same hospital.

Le Fort's data show that in lying-in hospitals in various countries and climates, scattered over nearly the whole of Europe, out of 888,312 deliveries there were no fewer than 30,394 deaths, giving an average death-rate of 34 per 1,000, a rate exceeding the high mortality which led to the discontinuance of our school for training midwifery nurses in King's College Hospital.

TABLE X. *Table Showing the Death-rate from all Causes amongst Women Delivered in Lying-in Hospitals.* (*Abstracted from Dr. Le Fort's ' Des Maternités.'*)

Maternity Hospitals	No. of Years of Observation	Deliveries	Deaths	Deaths per Thousand
Vienna Maternite . . .	50	103,731	2,811	25
Students' Clinique . .	30	104,492	5,560	53
Midwives „ . .	30	88,083	3,064	34
Académie Joséphine . .	1	277	24	86
Prague Maternité . . .	15	41,477	1,383	33
Munich „ . . .	4	4,064	86	21
Göttingen „ . . .	8	1,029	32	32
Gratz „ . . .	3	3,089	97	31
Greifswald Clinique . . .	4	316	18	56
Bremen Hospital . . .	6	139	10	71
Halle Clinique . . .	1	102	3	29
Berlin Clinique de l'Universite .	1	401	11	27
Frankfort-on-Main Maternite .	7	1,213	13	10
Leipzig Ancienne „ .	46	5,137	89	17
Nouvelle „ .	3	594	20	33
Pesth Clinique . . .	5	2,571	86	33
Moscow Maternité de la Maison des Enfans Trouvés . . .	11	11,556	230	19
Ditto	10	16,721	436	26
Ditto	10	27,759	776	28
St. Petersburg Clinique de la Faculte	6	376	34	90
Hospital Kalinkin .	15	1,288	20	15
Institut des Sages Femmes . .	15	8,036	238	29
Maternite des Enfans Trouvés . .	15	16,011	825	51
Dublin Maternite . . .	58	84,390	875	10
Ditto	7	21,867	309	14
Ditto	5	12,885	198	15
Ditto	7	16,391	158	9
Ditto	7	13,167	224	17
Ditto	7	13,699	179	13
Ditto	7	13,748	163	11
London Lying-in Hospital . .	28	5,883	172	29
Edinburgh Hospital . . .	1	277	3	10
Stuttgart „ . . .	1	424	3	7
Zurich Maternite . . .	1	200	20	100
Stockholm „ . . .	1	650	37	56
Göttenburg „ . . .	1	223	18	80
Lund „ . . .	1	33	2	60
Freiburg en Breisgau . .	3	281	10	35

C

Maternity Hospitals	No. of Years of Observation	Deliveries	Deaths	Deaths per Thousand
Jena Clinique . . .	4	308	21	67
Dresden Maternite . . .	51	15,356	373	27
Paris Maternite . . .	8	15,307	610	39
Ditto.	10	23,484	1,114	47
Ditto.	10	25,895	1,293	49
Ditto.	10	26,538	1,125	42
Ditto.	10	34,776	1,458	41
Ditto.	10	25,094	1,298	51
Ditto.	5	9,886	1,226	124
Total for ditto . . .	63	160,704	8,124	56
Paris Clinique de la Faculte .	5	1,654	117	70
Ditto.	10	9,079	359	39
Ditto.	10	9,462	379	40
Ditto.	5	4,100	288	70
Total for ditto . . .	30	24,295	1,143	47
Paris, St. Antoine . . .	9	28	5	178
Ditto.	10	32	15	468
Ditto.	10	129	20	155
Ditto.	10	788	65	82
Ditto.	10	2,359	134	56
Ditto.	5	1,868	110	58
Total for ditto . . .	54	5,204	349	67
Paris, Hôtel Dieu . . .	8	833	36	43
Ditto.	10	658	34	51
Ditto.	10	1,757	81	46
Ditto.	10	2,338	17	7
Ditto.	10	3,012	106	35
Ditto.	10	11,744	325	27
Ditto.	5	4,972	232	46
Total for ditto . . .	63	25,314	831	32
Paris, St. Louis . . .	3	4	0	0
Ditto.	10	128	2	15
Ditto.	10	1,282	51	39
Ditto.	10	2,832	173	61
Ditto.	10	2,736	102	37
Ditto.	10	7,244	200	27
Ditto.	5	3,812	252	66
Total for ditto . . .	58	19,038	780	40
Paris, La Charite . . .	3	648	84	126
Lyons „ . . .	4	3,325	91	17
Hôtel Dieu . .	4	2,016	33	16
Rouen Hôpital Général . .	4	1,275	9	7
Bordeaux Maternité . .	4	714	30	42
Lille	4	683	25	35
Rheims	4	646	15	23

Maternity Hospitals	No. of Years of Observation	Deliveries	Deaths	Deaths per Thousand
Strasburg	4	556	78	140
Grenoble	4	554	20	36
Bordeaux, St. Andre. . .	4	547	36	65
St. Etienne	4	515	8	15
Toulouse	4	493	9	18
Bourg	4	461	0	0
Troyes	4	460	2	4
Marseilles	4	444	16	36
Châteauroux. . . .	4	423	20	47
Amiens	4	396	5	12
Colmar	4	396	26	65
Nantes	4	340	17	50
Nancy	4	320	9	28
Orleans	4	301	3	9
Total for all hospitals . .	—	888,312	30,394	34

The absolute loss of life in Parisian lying-in wards has been greater than in those of any other capital city.

This is clearly shown in the 'Statistique medicale des Hopitaux de Paris,' kindly supplied to me by M. Husson, the Director of the General Administration of ' Public Assistance' at Paris, of whose many proofs of ability, activity, and benevolence, it is not here the place to speak. From this the following facts are abstracted. The death-rates are therein given for 12 hospitals receiving lying-in cases, only one of which, however, is a lying-in hospital (the ' Maison d'accouchement'), and will be found in Tables XI., XII., XIII.

In 1861 the average death-rate in these establishments was no less than 95.1 per 1,000.

In 1862 it was 69·7 per 1,000.

In 1863 it was 70·3 per 1,000.

TABLE XI.—*Mortality per Thousand among Lying-in Women at the undermentioned Parisian Hospitals during the Year* 1861. (*Abstracted from* '*Statistique Médicale des Hôpitaux*,' 1861.)

Hospital	Total Deliveries	Mortality per Thousand		
		Puerperal	Non-Puerperal	Total Deaths
Hotel Dieu . .	1,057	43·5	16·1	59·6
Pitie . . .	468	72·6	34·2	106·8
Charite . . .	253	154·2	39·7	193·7
St. Antoine . .	350	71·4	34·3	105·7
Necker . . .	234	29·9	29·9	59·8
Cochin . . .	56	142·9	35·7	178·6
Beaujon . . .	276	43·5	3·6	47·1
Lariboisière . .	782	69·1	15·3	84·4
St. Louis . . .	802	58·6	13·7	72·3
Lourcine . . .	41	24·4	—	24·4
Cliniques . . .	875	75·4	34·3	109·7
Maison d'Accouchements .	2,115	99·8	12·8	112·5
Total . .	7,309	75·2	19·8	95·1

TABLE XII.—*Mortality per Thousand among Lying-in Women at the undermentioned Parisian Hospitals during the Year* 1862. (*Abstracted from* '*Statistique Médicale des Hôpitaux de Paris*,' 1861, 2, 3.)

Hospital	Total Deliveries	Mortality per Thousand		
		Puerperal	Non-Puerperal	Total Deaths
Hôtel Dieu . . .	975	35·8	9·2	45·1
Pitié . . .	462	45·4	10·8	56·2
Charité . . .	270	62·9	25·9	88·8
St. Antoine . . .	311	61·0	19·2	80 3
Necker . . .	190	52·6	21·0	73·6
Cochin . . .	24	41·6	83·3	124·9
Beaujon . . .	257	38·9	19·9	58·8
Lariboisière . . .	816	34·3	13·5	47·8
St. Louis . . .	704	79·5	8·5	88·0
Lourcine . . .	45	22·2	—	22·2
Cliniques . . .	769	79·3	14·3	93·6
Maison d'Accouchements .	2,204	63·5	11·3	74·9
Total . .	7,027	56·7	12·9	69·7

TABLE XIII.—*Mortality per Thousand among Lying-in Women at the undermentioned Parisian Hospitals during the Year 1863. (Abstracted from ' Statistique Médicale des Hôpitaux,' 1863.)*

Hospital	Total Deliveries	Mortality per Thousand		
		Puerperal	Non-Puerperal	Total Deaths
Hôtel Dieu . . .	925	26·7	4·1	30·8
La Pitié . . .	544	44·1	1·8	46 0
Charite . . .	256	66·4	19·5	85·9
St. Antoine . . .	410	63·4	11·6	78·0
Necker . . .	232	38·8	21·6	60·3
Cochin . . .	68	73·5	14·7	88·2
Beaujon . . .	313	19·2	12·8	31·9
Lariboisière . . .	870	31·0	9·2	40·2
St. Louis . . .	871	23 0	9·2	32·1
Lourcine . . .	43	27·9	—	27·9
Clinique . . .	751	30·6	18·6	49·3
Maison d'Accouchements .	2,006	130·1	7·4	137·6
Total . .	7,289	60·6	9·7	70·3

CLASSIFICATION OF CAUSES OF MORTALITY IN LYING-IN INSTITUTIONS.

The next thing is to endeavour to show to what causes these death-rates are to be attributed. Unfortunately Dr. Le Fort's tables do not enable us to distinguish the causes of death. But the data supplied by British and Parisian hospitals allow the causes to be classified to a certain extent under the heads adopted by the Registrar-General in his Reports.

A classified arrangement of this kind is given in Table II., and may be resumed, with the view of showing the enormous differences in death-rates among puerperal women under different conditions, as follows :—

Mortality per 1,000.

	Puerperal diseases	Accidents of childbirth	Puerperal diseases and accidents of childbirth
All England, 13 years . . .	1·61	3·22	4·83
England (healthy districts), 10 years, 312,402 deliveries	—	—	4·3
England, 11 large towns, 10 years, 1,402,304 deliveries . . .	—	—	4·9
Liverpool workhouse . . .	3·4	2·2	5·6
27 London workhouses having deaths	4·1	2·1	6·2
8 military female hospitals . .	3·9	3·4	7·3
Queen Charlotte's Lying-in Hospital	14·3	5·3	19·6
King's College Hospital lying in ward	29·4	none	29·4
12 Parisian hospitals { 1861 . .	—	—	75·2
1862 . .	—	—	56·7
1863 . .	—	—	60·6

We have already seen, as a result of Dr. Le Fort's tables, that the mortality among women delivered at home, as deduced by him, is 4·7 per 1,000 ; while in the hospital it is 34 per 1,000, or nearly 7½-fold. Making any reasonable allowance for inaccuracy in the data, still we can hardly escape from his conclusions any more than we can rid ourselves from the consequences which follow from the data given above. We must confront the question called up by the data taken as a whole, viz., What can be the reason of this ascending scale of fatality shown on Table VIII. ? Why is it that these death-rates from all causes in childbirth, beginning at 5·1 per 1,000 for all England (town and country), successively become, among the same people 9·, 10·9, 14·3, 25·3, 33·3 ; and if we cross the channel, why should they mount up to 69, 70, and 95 per 1,000 ?

Again, why should fevers and inflammations of the puerperal class, which, as we have seen above, give a death-rate for all England of 1·61 per 1,000, mount up in English hospitals to 3·4, 4·1, 14·3, and 29·4 ? There must be some reason, besides the fact of childbirth, why diseases and accidents of this condition should be 4 times more fatal in a London lying-in hospital, and 15 times more fatal in Parisian hospitals, than they are in towns of England. What, then, are the immediate causes of these excessive death-rates ?

CAUSES OF HIGH DEATH-RATES IN LYING-IN INSTITUTIONS.

The determining causes of these death-rates need to be discussed most cautiously ;—our information concerning them being so scanty.

We know from Statistics that these Deaths occur, but why they occur and why they vary are questions not yet to be fully answered in our present stage of knowledge (or of ignorance).

At one time a sufficient cause seems to present itself; but the very next outbreak of Puerperal disease may occur under quite different conditions. For years an Institution may escape excessive Mortality ; and then it may suffer severely under the same apparent circumstances. All that we can do at present is to see whether there are removable causes in cases where the Mortality is excessive, and to remove them. Fully recognising how much we have need ot caution, this subject will be next considered generally and as far as possible in its practical bearings on the points at issue.

There are some important remarks in Dr. Le Fort's book, bearing on this subject, which may find a place here.

Puerperal Fever.—Dr. Le Fort states, as the result of his enquiry, that the frequency of obstetrical operations modifies the general mortality only in a slight degree; that the excessive mortality in lying-in hospitals is much greater than can be attributed to ordinary hospital influences; that it depends neither on the social condition of the women, nor on the moral conditions under which delivery may occur; that it may be more or less influenced by the insalubrity of particular hospitals, but that puerperal fever is the principal cause of death after delivery; that this disease shows itself in all hospitals, in all maternity institutions, in all climates, in the south of France as it does at St. Petersburg, in Dublin as in Vienna, in London as in Moscow. It exists in America as in Europe.

It is less frequent and fatal during the summer months, attributable in part at least to greater facilities of ventilation following on higher temperature (in other words, to having your windows open instead of shut).

This disease develops itself spontaneously under certain unknown circumstances. When it is about to become epidemic, it is sometimes preceded by the prevalence of erysipelas.

Dr. Le Fort points out that what was considered a severe epidemic in the British Lying-in Hospital, in the year 1770, is ' unfortunately less than the *mean* mortality of the Maternite at Paris.'

While admitting that puerperal fever may originate *de novo*, Dr. Le Fort dwells strongly on the communicability of the disease as an efficient cause of its prevalence.

He adduces opinions of the following physicians—Oppolzer, Rokitansky, and Skoda, of Vienna ; Virchow, of Berlin ; Lange, of Heidelberg ; Schwarz, of Gottingen ; Loschner, of Prague ; and Hecker, of Munich—on the nature and origin of this fatal disease. Generally they testify to the propagation of puerperal fever by contagion, but they also state that it is a blood disease—a product of foul air, putrid miasms, and predisposition to malignant inflammatory action.

Dr. Le Fort also cites a number of interesting facts, showing that the indiscriminate visiting by attendants of lying-in women and patients suffering from disease, either within or outside the same establishment, has been a means of exciting puerperal fever action.

Admission of Students.—It is one of the contingencies necessarily due to connecting together the teaching of midwifery to students, with other portions of clinical instruction, that no precautions can prevent a student passing from a bad surgical case, or from an anatomical theatre, to the bedside of a lying-in woman, while sad experience has proved that the most fatal results may ensue from this circumstance.

Of course risks of this kind are greatly increased when

there are lying-in wards in general hospitals—especially if a medical school be attached to such a hospital.

This risk had not been overlooked in the arrangements for the lying-in wards at King's College Hospital, under which, while intended solely for the training of midwifery nurses, provision was made for a limited and regulated attendance of students; but, when enquiries came to be made into the probable cause of the high death-rates, it was found that the restrictions laid down as to the admission of students had been disregarded; also that there was a post-mortem theatre almost under the ward windows.

Effect of Numbers.—Dr. Le Fort has examined the influence exercised by numbers—or, in other words, by the size of hospitals—on the mortality after childbirth. His general results may be briefly stated as follows :—

In hospitals receiving annually more than 2,000 lying-in cases, comprising the two Cliniques of Vienna, 1834–63; the Maternites of Paris, 1849–59; of Prague, 1848–62; and of Moscow, 1853–62; and the Lying-in Hospital of Dublin, 1847–54, the death-rate is 40·7 per 1,000.

In hospitals receiving between 1,000 and 2,000 cases a year, including the Enfans Trouves at Petersburg, 1845–59; the Maternite at Munich, 1859–62, and other places, the death-rate is 36 per 1,000.

In hospitals receiving from 500 to 1,000 cases a year, including Pesth and the Maternite of Dresden, the death-rate is nearly 27 per 1,000.

In hospitals where the number of deliveries is between 200 and 500 per annum, comprehending several places cited, among the rest Edinburgh and the London Lying-in Hospital, 1833–60, the death-rate is 30½ per 1,000.

In hospitals receiving between 100 and 200 cases, as at Frankfort and Gottingen, the death-rate is 27·6 per 1,000.

And in three small establishments receiving fewer than 100 a-year, as at Lund, the death-rate is above 83½ per 1,000.

From these facts Dr. Le Fort concludes that the relative mortality in small and large establishments is not favourable to small hospitals, *per se.* The benefit of subdivision may be neutralised by other circumstances.

We must also protest against massing hospitals, alike only in one circumstance, together for the sake of taking their statistics *in bulk* in this way, except for the most general purposes—which is indeed all Dr. Le Fort has in view here —especially as our own lying-in institutions of these islands, which come out best individually, appear here confounded amongst the greatest sinners. But Dr. Le Fort's general conclusion, against the influence of size *per se,* is no doubt correct.

As a general rule, statistics appear to show that the great mortality of lying-in hospitals is of periodical occurrence.

Puerperal women, as everyone knows, are the most susceptible of all subjects to ' blood-poisoning.' The smallest transference of putrescing miasm from a locality where such miasm exists to the bedside of a lying-in patient is most dangerous. Puerperal women are, moreover, exposed to the risks of ' blood-poisoning ' by the simple fact of being brought together in lying-in wards, and especially by being retained a longer time than is absolutely necessary in lying-in wards after being delivered, while to a great extent they escape this entire class of risks by being attended at home.

There are no doubt difficulties in assigning the exact effect of every condition to which a lying-in woman may be exposed in contributing to these death-rates, but there are, nevertheless, a few great fundamental facts which arrest attention in such an enquiry.

It is a fact, for instance, that however grand, or however humble, a home may be in which the birth of a child takes place, there is only one delivery in the home at one time. Another fact is, that a second delivery will certainly not take place in the same room, inhabited by the same couple, for 10 months at least, and may not take place in the same room for years. The Registrar-General has shown us that under these conditions the death-rate among lying-in women all over England, and from all registered causes, is about 5·1 per 1,000.

In many London workhouses the number of deliveries yearly is so small that, so far as concerns annual deliveries, they approach more closely to dwelling-houses divided among a number of families than they do to lying-in hospitals properly so called.

Let us now see what relation there is between the annual deliveries and the death-rates in these workhouse wards.

Assuming that the London workhouse lying-in wards have certain conditions in common, we find that twenty-seven infirmaries suffered from lying-in deaths in five years, and that in thirteen there were no deaths in the same years. Now, in each of these twenty-seven hospitals yielding deaths, the deliveries averaged 29 per annum, while in the thirteen infirmaries without deaths the deliveries averaged under 16 per annum.

Again, in twenty-one infirmaries with deaths, the average disposable space for each occupied lying-in bed was 2,246 cubic feet; while in nine infirmaries without deaths the space per occupied bed averaged 3,149 cubic feet. These, however, are only averages, and as such may be taken for what they are worth. There were exceptions to these rules in particular cases.

The facts regarding Waterford Lying-in Institution have a very important bearing on this question of subdivision.

In the years from 1838 to 1844 this hospital consisted of two rooms in a small house. One room was a delivery ward. The other held eight lying-in beds. The total deliveries in this house amounted to 753, and there were 6 deaths = 8 per 1,000. Half this mortality was due to puerperal fever.

In October 1844 this hospital occupied another small house, in which the eight lying-in beds were placed in two rooms instead of one as formerly — four beds per room. Up to October 1867 there had been 2,656 deliveries in this house, and 9 deaths — a mortality of 3·4 per 1,000. There were only two puerperal fever deaths in these 2,656 deliveries.

These facts appear to show that subdivision among lying-in cases has a certain influence in warding off mortality.

But, on the other hand, the death-rates among lying-in

cases in particular hospitals are not always in the ratio of the number of occupied beds. A few illustrations of this will suffice.

Thus, in the year 1861, there were in the Rotunda Hospital, Dublin, 1,135 deliveries, on which the death-rate was 51·9 per 1,000. In 1828 the deliveries were 2,856, and the death-rate 15 per 1,000. In the four years 1830 to 1833, the deliveries varied from 2,138 to 2,288, and the death-rates were a little more than 5 per 1,000. In Queen Charlotte's Hospital the highest death-rate occurred in 1849, during which year there were 161 deliveries. The death-rate was 93·2 per 1,000, while in 1832, with 217 deliveries, the death-rate was just one tenth of this amount.

In the Maison d'Accouchement at Paris, during the five decennial periods between 1810 and 1859,[1] there were 141,476 deliveries, among which there occurred 6,288 deaths, giving a death-rate of 44·4 per 1,000. The lowest death rate in any of the decennial periods occurred between 1840 and 1849, when it amounted to 41·9 per 1,000. The largest number of deliveries of any period in the half century was during this ten years. They amounted to 34,776; while, in the period from 1850 to 1859, the deliveries were 24,944, and the death-rate 52 per 1,000.

The Dublin Rotunda approximates most to this Paris Maternite in the large number of deliveries, vibrating around 2,000 a year; while, in Queen Charlotte's Hospital,

---

[1] Husson, ' Etude sur les Hopitaux,' p. 254.

where, even since its reconstruction, the mortality has been in many years higher than in the Dublin Rotunda, the number of annual deliveries has varied around 200.

Danger of Puerperal Epidemics.—These facts have a very important bearing on the whole question of lying-in institutions, for they show that, with scarcely an exception, while the lowest death-rate in any given year greatly exceeds the average mortality among lying-in women delivered at home, the inmates of these institutions are exposed to the enormous additional risk of puerperal epidemics.

Take, for instance, Queen Charlotte's Hospital. There is no reason to believe that less care and solicitude for the welfare of its inmates is exercised than would be the case if they were delivered at home. And yet we find that year by year, from 1828 down to the present time, the institution has only escaped deaths for four years. The lowest death-rate it ever had was in 1835, when it amounted to 4·6 per 1,000. In other years it has been 11, 15, 21, 30, 50, 70, 81, 86, and in one year it rose to the immense death-rate of 93·2 per 1,000.

In 1849 there were, as above said, 161 deliveries out of which fourteen women died from puerperal fever, being a death-rate of 87 per 1,000 from this disease alone.

The statistics of other lying-in institutions afford corresponding data. It is a lamentable fact that the mortality in lying-in wards from childbirth, which is *not* a disease, approaches closely to the mortality from all diseases and accidents together in general hospitals, and in many instances even greatly exceeds this mortality. It is the more lamentable, because, as need scarcely be stated, the causes of a higher mortality in infancy and old age cannot exist at child-bearing ages. Also, childbirth ought certainly not to be a 'miasmatic disease.' Unless, then, it can be clearly shown that these enormous death-rates can be abated, or that they are altogether inevitable, does not the whole of the evidence with regard to special lying-in hospitals lead but to one conclusion, viz. that they should be closed? Is there any conceivable amount of privation which would warrant such a step as bringing together a constant number of puerperal women into the same room, in buildings constructed and managed on the principles embodied in existing lying-in institutions?

Fatality of Lying-in Wards in General Hospitals.—Besides special lying-in hospitals, there are general hospitals which receive lying-in cases. Fortunately, there are not many such in England. But in Paris there are 11[1] general hospitals which receive midwifery cases. A reference to Tables XI., XII., XIII., will show how great the risks are to lying-in women under the same roof with medical and surgical cases; a fact which may be further illustrated by a reference to data for particular hospitals. For example, in 1861, 253 lying-in cases in La Charite gave a total death-rate of 193·7 per 1,000, of which no less than 154·2 was due to puerperal causes. These tables tell their own story,

[1] Tables XI., XII., XIII., abstracted from the 'Statistique médicale des Hopitaux de Paris.'

and they throw altogether into the shade the lamentable losses at King's College Hospital.

The only *amende* that could be made was to shut up the ward ; and having done this in the interest of womankind, need it be said that the impression produced by these statistics confirms the conclusion just stated in regard to existing lying-in wards generally, and is that not a single lying-in woman should ever pass within the doors of a general hospital ? Is not any risk which can be incurred outside almost infinitely smaller ? And as a general hospital must always be a hospital, must not this verdict be an absolute one, not one which can be altered or reversed ?

INFLUENCE OF CONSTRUCTION AND MANAGEMENT OF LYING-IN WARDS ON THE DEATH-RATE.

Before, however, surrendering entirely the principle of special lying-in institutions, it is only fair to enquire whether the construction, management, and arrangements of existing hospitals of this class may possibly have had any influence upon the mortality, apart from the mere fact of bringing lying-in cases together under one roof.

This question is the more important because we now know that construction and arrangement of buildings exert a notable effect on the death statistics of general hospitals. It is at last universally admitted that airy open site, simplicity of plan, subdivision of cases under a number of separate pavilions, large cubic space, abundant fresh air, mainly from windows on the opposite sides of the wards, drainage arrange-

ments entirely outside the hospital, are essential conditions
to the safety of all general hospitals. But, as already stated,
it is likewise admitted that lying-in women are peculiarly
susceptible to ' blood poisoning.'

This being the case, have we any reason to expect other
than a high death-rate if we collect lying-in women into
such wards, or rather rooms, as are found in many old hos
pitals ?

Nobody with ordinary knowledge of the subject, and
desirous simply of benefiting suffering people, would now
dream of appropriating buildings of this kind as hospitals
for sick. But it is to be feared that the same scruple
has not always existed with regard to lying-in women.
And as we now know that such buildings give high death-
rates among sick and wounded people, there is every reason
to fear that they have had their share in raising the death-
rate among lying-in women to a greater extent than that
due merely to the fact of agglomeration. As instances of
the existence of danger from such causes, and also from
grave errors in administration, two or three illustrations
are here introduced from existing lying-in establishments.

Maternité, Paris.—We have seen from the statistics that
the chief of chief offenders in times past has been the
Maternité at Paris. This establishment was in former
times the monastery of ' Port Royal de Paris.' It is situated in one of the most healthy open spots on the outskirts
of the French capital, and, as far as situation is concerned,
ought to be healthy. The building was devoted to its
present destination in 1795, and has undergone many

changes since that date. It contains 228 beds for lying-in women, and, besides, accommodation for 94 pupil midwives. From 1,000 to 2,200 deliveries and upwards take place here annually : from 1840 to 1849 there were as many as 3,400 annually. Until recently it consisted properly of three divisions, delivery wards, cells for delivered women in the process of recovery, and an infirmary.

The delivery ward is well lighted on two sides, and communicates with an operation theatre, where lectures are also given.

The woman, if progressing favourably after delivery, was removed to one of the cells in what may be called the recovery ward. The construction of these cells was as follows :—a long corridor, with windows on opposite sides, was divided into separate cells, each cell having its own window, by partitions stretching one third across the corridor, but not cut off on the end towards the middle of the corridor. Each cell was provided with a bed and a cradle, so that in walking up the centre of the corridor the divisions, or rather the cells, opened right and left from the passage, like the stalls of a stable. This construction rendered it almost impossible to open the windows. The infirmary consisted of small wards of three or four beds each, into which were moved indiscriminately patients suffering with all classes of disease. And it appears, from Dr. Le Fort's account, that pupil midwives had at the same time patients in the infirmary, and healthy women, both delivered and not delivered, under their care. Pregnant women are often admitted weeks, and even months delivery, at the Maternite. [So also at the Midwives' Clinique at Vienna.]

Recently the cells have been removed from the corridor, and glass partitions have been thrown across from back to front, each division containing six beds, but communicating with the adjoining divisions by means of doors intended to be used only when the service requires it.

The infirmary has been completely separated from this portion of the establishment, but all classes of cases are still transferred into the infirmary as before.

As consequences of these arrangements, we have in the Maternité the following conditions :—

1. The agglomeration of a number of lying-in women under the same roof.

2. An internal construction of the building not suited to give fresh air, to say the least of it.

3. The infirmary until recently connected with the other portions of the building, and even now receiving all classes of cases among lying-in women, whether febrile or not, for treatment.

4. One class of attendants devoted indiscriminately to all classes of inmates.

5. As already mentioned, women admitted and retained within the walls of the establishment before and after the time simply required for delivery and convalescence.

Lastly, an enormous death-rate mainly from puerperal diseases.

Hôpital de la Clinique, Paris.—This establishment is part of the hospital for clinical instruction, close to the buildings of the Ecole de Medecine. The hospital consists of a parallelogram with a central court, containing not only the clinical surgery wards, but also an amphitheatre devoted to anatomical studies, with a mean number of fifty corpses in the course of dissection.

There are six wards devoted to the midwifery department, arranged in a complicated manner, partly across the corridor, and partly on each side of the corridor, all of them entered from a central passage lighted by the open doors of the wards along the sides. They contained 54 lying-in beds. From 800 to 900 deliveries took place here annually. 18 to 20 days appear to be the average stay. The beds must, therefore, have been pretty constantly full.

The wards devoted to women who have been delivered communicate freely with one another by open doors. The beds are curtained, and the curtains are washed only once in six months, even though the occupants of the bed may have died of puerperal fever. The beds are of iron, and are provided with a spring mattress, over which is a wool mattress. The latter is removed after each delivery, cleansed, and renewed. There is no infirmary for diseases ; whether cases of puerperal fever or others, all are treated in the beds in which they are placed after delivery.

The female staff performs its duty to all classes of cases.

Students entered upon the roll for midwifery practice are called into the wards from other parts of the establishment by signals placed in a window.

It is quite unnecessary to search for any more recondite

causes of the past excessive mortality of this establishment than these simple facts.

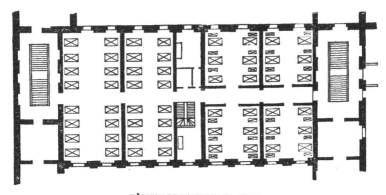

HÔPITAL DE LA CLINIQUE, PARIS.

(*Former arrangement of Lying-in Wards.*)

The above plan, taken from M. Husson's 'Etude sur les Hôpitaux,' will show the arrangement of wards and beds in this place. [Dr. Le Fort says that the number of beds in each ward has since been reduced by a third.]

Queen Charlotte's Lying-in Hospital, London.—Plate I. shows a plan and section of Queen Charlotte's Hospital, as rebuilt in 1856.

On each floor are 6 wards, containing 3 beds each, in which the patients are delivered, with an average of 1,000 cubic feet to each patient. On each floor, also, is one convalescent ward, containing 6 beds. Two floors are devoted to patients : one for married, and one for single women. As soon as 3 patients have been delivered in a ward, it remains vacant for 8 or 10 days, and is cleansed. Patients are removed as soon as possible to the convalescent ward.

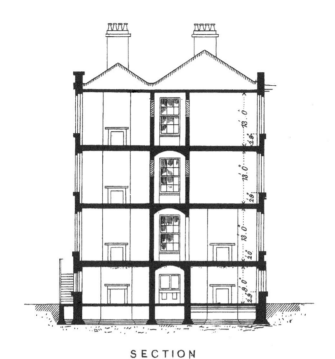

SECTION

Queen Charlottes Lying in Hospital

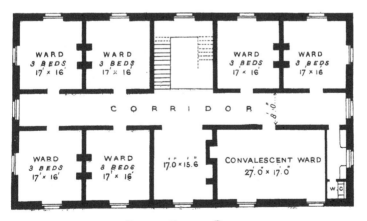

| WARD 3 BEDS 17 × 16 | WARD 3 BEDS 17 × 16 | | WARD 3 BEDS 17 × 16 | WARD 3 BEDS 17 × 16 |

C O R R I D O R

| WARD 3 BEDS 17 × 16 | WARD 3 BEDS 17 × 16 | 17.0 × 15.6 | CONVALESCENT WARD 27.0 × 17.0 |

W.C

FIRST FLOOR PLAN.

Scale

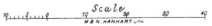

10   10   20   30   40

M & N. HANHART LITH.

When a case of fever occurs, the ward is freshly white-washed, and not occupied again for at least a month.

In this building we have three floors and a basement. A drain runs from back to front of the building, right across the basement—a most unsafe course for a drain in any inhabited building.[1]

It will be seen that the rooms are placed on opposite sides of a main corridor running the lengthway of the building on each floor; that the corridors of the different floors communicate by the stairs; that the ventilation of each room communicates with the ventilation of every other room through the corridors; that none of the rooms have windows on opposite sides, and that there are water-closets having a ventilation common to that of the building. Now every one of these structural arrangements is objectionable, and would be considered so in any good hospital, and nobody now-a-days would venture to include all of them in a general hospital plan. They are hence *à fortiori* altogether inadmissible in a building for the reception of lying-in women.

We have thus, in Queen Charlotte's Hospital, the following defects :—

1. Agglomeration of a number of cases under the same roof.

2. A form of construction unsuited for hospital purposes.

3. No means of removing outside the building febrile or other cases of puerperal diseases from the vicinity of patients recovering after delivery.

[1] This drain was shown on the Plan from which Plate I. is taken.

Since 1856, notwithstanding the great improvements, the death-rates per 1,000 have been 12·2, 8·8, 81·2, 70·3, 54·2, 39·2, 15·5, and so on : in several years very considerably larger than the mortality which led to the closing of the lying-in wards in King's College Hospital. These varying deaths lead to the exercise of much caution in drawing conclusions as to their causes ; but the main fact remains, namely, there are the death-rates, and they are many times greater than occur among London poor women delivered at home.

Midwifery Wards, King's College Hospital.—The following plan shows the provision which existed for training midwifery nurses at King's College Hospital.

MIDWIFERY WARDS, KING'S COLLEGE HOSPITAL.
(Plan of Third Floor.)

A, A. Accouchement Wards, used alternately.
B. Recovery Ward.
C. Contains Linen Presses, and Infants' Baths, &c., for Ward use.
D. Superior's Bed-room.
E. Midwife's Room.
F. Post-mortem Theatre.
G, G. General and Provision Hoists.

K. This roof is not higher than the basement.
×. Ventilating openings on a level with upper part of opposite window.
a, a, a, a. Doors cutting off communication with either Accouchement Ward when necessary.
b. No. 4 Ward.

The plan shows the relation of the delivery wards to the recovery ward, and to the other parts of the hospital; to the lecture room, post mortem theatre, &c. The main defects in the construction are : the back to back wards; proximity of these wards to the general wards of the hospital; the large staircase, common to both sets of wards, although its size and openness, and the windows opposite each other and on each floor, ensured ventilation, and separated the respective blocks; the position of the post-mortem theatre, the smell from which, as stated on the best authority, could be distinctly detected in the wards. As already stated, students were admitted from other parts of the hospital to the midwifery wards.

RESULTS OF IMPROVED LYING-IN WARD CONSTRUCTION.

A few instances of improved lying in ward construction, together with the death-rates in these establishments, will next be given.

Military Female Hospitals.—These buildings vary in constructive arrangements. Some are much better than others, and during recent years lying-in wards of improved construction have been provided in connection with several newly erected military female hospitals. The earlier plans of the new female hospitals consist of a block formed of two pavilions joined end to end, with a passage across the block to separate the pavilions from each other. Each pavilion contains a single ward, with its own separate offices and nurses' rooms. It has windows on opposite sides, with one large end window, and abundant means of warming and ventilation. One pavilion is devoted to general cases, the other to lying-in cases.

The midwifery ward has space for twelve beds. Each bed has a superficial area of ninety square feet, and a cubic space of 1,350 feet. The wards are fifteen feet high.

Two hospitals on this plan have been in use at Woolwich and Chatham for upwards of six years. During this period there have been at the two 1,093 deliveries, and 11 deaths. At Chatham there was one accidental death from removal of the patient to hospital, and out of 342 deliveries there have been no deaths from puerperal diseases. There were, however, two deaths from scarlet fever, occurring while this disease was prevalent in soldiers' families in the garrison. At Woolwich, among 751 deliveries, there have been 8 deaths, of which five were from puerperal diseases, but of these five deaths one took place in a woman who had gastric fever at the time of admission, and in other two women puerperal peritonitis came on after instrumental delivery. There was one death from embolism, one from exhaustion, and one from dropsy. The total death-rate in these two hospitals has been under 10 per 1,000. The deaths due to diseases and accidents of childbirth have been 6, or at the rate of $5\frac{1}{2}$ per 1,000.

Of the other military hospitals, the statistics of which are given in Table IV., Devonport and Portsmouth are unsuitable adapted buildings. Aldershot Hospital consists of a number of huts joined together as a general female hospital, with accommodation for all kinds of cases, including lying-in cases. This arrangement is a very undesirable one, and the results have been unsatisfactory.

Table XIV. shows that the total mortality in this hospital has been 10·1 per 1,000. Of the total deaths 27 are attributed to diseases and accidents of childbirth, affording a mortality of 8·8 per 1,000, or double that of the healthy districts of England.

If we exclude Aldershot as being unfit for child-birth cases, we find that in the other seven hospitals the total mortality, as shown in Table XIV., has been 7·4 per 1,000. The mortality from puerperal diseases in these hospitals has been 2·7 per 1,000, and from diseases and accidents of childbirth 5·4 per 1,000.

TABLE XIV.

	All Women's Hospitals (Military)					Aldershot Women's Hospital					Other Women's Hospitals, excluding Aldershot				
	Puerperal Diseases	Accidents of Childbirth	Diseases and Accidents of Childbirth	Others	Total Mortality	Puerperal Diseases	Accidents of Childbirth	Diseases and Accidents of Childbirth	Others	Total Mortality	Puerperal Diseases	Accidents of Childbirth	Diseases and Accidents of Childbirth	Others	Total Mortality
Deaths per 1,000 deliveries	3·9	3·4	7·3	1·5	8·8	4·9	3·9	8·8	1·3	10·1	2·7	2·7	5·4	2·0	7·4

There are two camp hospitals for lying-in cases, consisting only of wooden huts, appropriated for the purpose, which have yielded very important experience. One of these is at Colchester, the other at Shorncliffe.

The Shorncliffe Hospital is an old wooden hut of the simplest construction, with thorough ventilation. It is situated on a rising ground close to the sea, and facing it, so that the sea breeze sweeps right through it. It is scarcely more than a makeshift. And here are the results.

Table IV. shows that up to December 1869, there had been 702 deliveries in the hut, among which there was one death from scarlet fever, and one from hæmorrhage, besides two deaths following on craniotomy. There was not a single death from any puerperal disease.

Colchester Lying-in Hospital, of which a plan and section are given on Plate II., is nothing more than an ordinary officer's wooden hut, divided by partitions into four compartments, with a transverse passage cutting them off from each other. This hut has been in use for a considerable number of years as a place of lying-in for soldiers' wives living in the camp, and there have been altogether between 500 and 600 deliveries in it. The matron states that during the whole time the hut has been in use for its present purpose, no death has taken place in it. But as statistics have only been kept since 1865, we shall limit our attention to them. They show that, up to the end of October 1870, there had been 252 registered deliveries, and no deaths.

The results of these two makeshift hospitals, when compared with the figures already given for lying-in establishments generally, are certainly remarkable. They are both detached buildings, having no connection with any general hospital. Their construction ensures a plentiful supply of fresh air at all times. They contain very few beds, and these beds are occupied, seldom or never, all at one time. Indeed, it is stated that in the Colchester hut there is scarcely more than one, or at most two beds, constantly

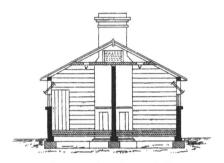

SECTION ON LINE A.B

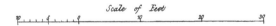

Scale of Feet

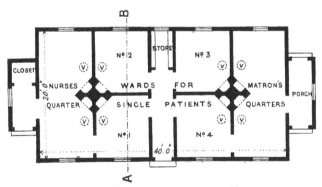

PLAN OF WOODEN LYING IN HUT
COLCHESTER CAMP

v. *Foul air outlets.*

occupied throughout the year. Also, soldiers' wives lying-in rarely remain more than ten days, though sometimes twelve in hospital. There is, therefore, no crowding; scrupulous cleanliness is observed; there are no sources of putrid miasm in or near the lying-in huts; and they have their own attendants. The data in Table IV. show that there have been 954 registered deliveries in the two huts, and four deaths, of which three were due to puerperal accidents, and none to puerperal diseases.

PROPOSED HOSPITAL FOR WOMEN, PORTSMOUTH.

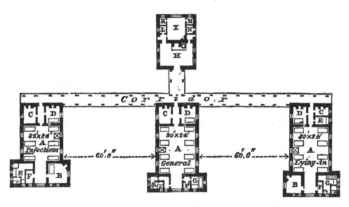

PLAN.

A. Wards.	F. Linen.	L. Medical Comforts.
B. Spare Wards.	G. Baths.	M. Store.
C. Sculleries.	H. Kitchen.	N. Coals.
D. Nurses.	I. Cook's Room.	
E. Lavatories.	K. Store.	

Proposed new Female Hospital at Portsmouth.—When military female hospitals were first designed, it was intended that they should receive only lying-in and general cases from married soldiers' families in separate pavilions. But at a subsequent date zymotic cases were admitted into the same pavilion with general cases. Very decided objections were, however, urged against this step by medical officers, and the next hospital planned was divided into three distinct pavilions. It was intended for Portsmouth garrison, and is shown in the annexed figure.

A female hospital on this plan has been erected at Dublin, with the two end wards built in the line of the corridor beyond the ends of it, in place of at right angles to the corridor, as shown in the proposed Portsmouth plan. By this form of construction the cases received from soldiers' families can be divided into three classes: general, infectious, and midwifery—each class in its own separate building. Such, however, has been the feeling of medical officers as to the undesirableness of trusting even to this amount of separation, that at Dublin the 'infectious' cases have been removed to another locality altogether. The same separation had been already effected at Chatham and Woolwich.

Close observation of lying-in cases has led to further change in the construction, and it is now proposed to adopt for lying-in wards in female hospitals a different form of arrangement altogether : namely, to divide the lying-in pavilion into separate one-bed rooms, as shown on Plan IV.

The experience of these small military female lying-in hospitals has shown the favourable effect of simplicity of construction, plenty of space, light, and fresh air, perfect cleanliness, a small number of lying-in beds, not by any means constantly occupied, administration separate from that of general hospitals, and allowing the lying-in women to return to quarters in as few days after delivery as their recovery admits.

But there is one remarkable instance in which a plan of construction, on the principle of the earlier British military female hospitals described above, has been adopted without having led to equally satisfactory results.

The new 'Maternité' belonging to the Hôpital Cochin at Paris has been constructed on a ground-plan similar to that at Woolwich, viz., with two pavilions projecting in line from a centre, and containing two ten-bed wards. It is in two floors, with small wards on the upper floor. Part of its sanitary arrangements are certainly not what we should adopt in this country, but there are many hospitals in which there are worse defects.

Puerperal fever appeared in this hospital within a month of its being opened.

Where so much attention had been paid to construction, the causes of the fever must be looked for somewhere else than in the ward plan.

Dr. Le Fort has stated that puerperal fever cases had been retained temporarily in the wards after the development of the disease; that the same nurses took charge, not only of cases of disease in the isolated wards, but also of women making healthy recoveries; and that there is nothing to prevent the medical attendant passing almost directly from the autopsy of a puerperal fever case to render assistance to a healthy woman.

This experience is very important. It shows how much the safety of lying-in hospitals depends on common-sense management, and that it would be disastrous to trust to improved construction alone, while everything else is left to take its own course.

We now arrive at the consideration of an elementary point :—

SHOULD MEDICAL STUDENTS BE ADMITTED TO LYING-IN HOSPITAL PRACTICE?

This is a very grave question. Medical students were admitted to the lying-in wards at King's College Hospital. Was this one cause of the occurrence of puerperal diseases there?

There are facts, it is true, such as those supplied by the Maternité and Clinique at Paris (the latter only admitting medical students), in both of which establishments the mortality is excessive, which on first sight appear to show that the presence of medical students in a lying-in hospital is not necessarily a cause of adding to a mortality already excessive. But on the other hand there are facts, such as those given by Dr. Le Fort, admitting of a comparison being made between the mortality in lying-in wards to which medical students are admitted with the mortality in other wards of the same establishment not admitting students, which appear to establish the point conclusively. The special case he cites is the following :—

At Vienna there are two lying-in cliniques, one for students and one for midwives. They are both situated in the same hospital, and their external conditions are insufficient in themselves to explain the facts now to be noted. Puerperal fever prevailed in the hospital during the same months in ten separate years, from 1838 to 1862, and the following table gives the mortality per 1,000 in each set of clinical wards :—

| YEARS | MONTHS | MORTALITY PER 1,000 | |
		1st Clinique Students	2nd Clinique Midwives
1838	June	9	247
1839	July	150	34
1840	October	293	58
1842	December	313	37
1844	November	170	33
1844	March	110	7
1845	October	148	13
1846	May	134	4
1847	April	179	7
1856	September	13	105
1862	December	63	2

Is it not quite clear that some bad influence was at work in this case on the students' side, which was not in force on the pupil midwives' side? That there was something else in operation besides epidemic influence is shown by the much greater frequency and severity of puerperal diseases in the one clinique than in the other. We may assume the fact without attempting to explain it, as a proof of the necessity of separating midwifery instruction altogether from ordinary hospital clinical instruction; and does not this Vienna history throw fresh light on the experience already alluded to of our midwives' school in King's College Hospital?

E

*INFLUENCE OF TIME SPENT IN A LYING-IN WARD
ON THE DEATH-RATE.*

This very important element in the question of mortality
has been already referred to.   There appear to be no
extant statistics to show the relation of the death-rate to the
period of residence.   This much, however, is known—that in
the establishments where the death rate is highest the probable effect of length of residence appears not to be considered, while in the cases cited where the death-rates are
lowest the women leave the hospital as soon as they are able
to do so.

Dr. Le Fort, however, quotes Tarnier and Lasserre of
Paris, and Späth of Vienna, as holding that the death-rate is
lower among women admitted some time before labour.
'They become acclimatised' (an odd expression, when
applied to the foul air of an establishment where there
should be no foul air).   He also says that puerperal fever is
very rare among women brought into hospital *after* delivery,
and he asks whether 'contamination does not take place
principally and almost solely at the moment of accouchement.'

One can only repeat, what indeed Le Fort states, that in
these most important points of enquiry, the very elements
are yet wanting to us.

Some hospitals have rather plumed themselves on their
humanity in giving shelter to poor lying-in women as long
as possible, while in military lying-in hospitals soldiers'
wives are obliged to go home as soon as they can, to help
the domestic earnings.   In the first class the death-rate is
high, in the last it is low.

The low death-rates in workhouse lying-in wards appear

to support this conclusion also. These do not retain together women not yet in labour, women in labour, women delivered, and convalescent women. Their principle, on the contrary, is to receive women when labour is imminent, and to send them out of the ward as speedily as possible.

A moment's consideration will be sufficient to show how important a point in management this is. If there is any danger at all to puerperal women in a lying-in institution (a fact which has been proved), is it not clear that the danger must become cumulative? It will increase in a certain ratio as the length of residence increases.

Blood-poisoning, if once begun, will not stop of itself unless the subject of it be removed from the cause, or the cause from the subject, if it stop even then. To retain both subject and cause together is simply to render certain that which under better management might have been evanescent. The more this question is considered the more important does it appear, as involving an element exercising a very considerable influence on the ultimate fate of inmates of lying-in institutions. The institution, by retaining its inmates, becomes a hospital ; and, as such, subjects its inmates to hospital influences while in the most susceptible of all conditions.

The absence of information in almost all published statistics on the point would be grotesque, if it were not alarming from the carelessness it shows. With some difficulty the following few meagre data have been scraped together as to the average number of days lying-in women spend in the undermentioned institutions :—

Soldiers' Wives' Hospitals	10 to 12 days
Liverpool Workhouse Lying-in Wards .	14 ,,
London Workhouse Lying-in Wards . .	14, 18, 21 ,,
Paris Maternité	17, 18 ,,
Paris Clinique	18, 20 ,,
King's College Hospital	16 ,,

This involves the question of management, which is next to be considered.

EFFECT OF GOOD MANAGEMENT ON THE SUCCESS OF LYING-IN ESTABLISHMENTS.

The most important experience which can be had as to the effect of good management in preventing the development of puerperal diseases is afforded by the results of midwifery cases in workhouse infirmaries. In none of these institutions is there any great refinement of construction or of sanitary appliances, and nevertheless their death-rates have been much lower than those of maternity institutions generally.

In Table V. are given the statistics of the lying-in wards of Liverpool workhouse for thirteen years. During this period there were an approximate number of 6,396 deliveries and 58 deaths, giving a total death-rate of 9·06 per 1,000.

Of these deaths 22 were from puerperal diseases —equal to a death-rate of 3·4 per 1,000. There were 14 deaths from accidents of childbirth—equal to a death-rate of 2·2 per 1,000. The aggregate death-rate from puerperal diseases and accidents of childbirth was 5·6 per 1,000.

These deaths are said to include all among puerperal women delivered in these lying-in wards, whether occurring within or without the maternity division. Mr. Barnes, the medical officer of the establishment, states that he can 'answer for this with certainty' during the last 5 years. Also, that no lying-in woman is discharged out of the workhouse unless in perfect health, so that no puerperal death can have happened after discharge. Mr. Barnes has farther been kind enough to supply data for the following 3 years' statistics, to show the general character of the cases which have furnished these low death-rates.

Summary of Cases Delivered in the Lying-in Wards of Liverpool Workhouse 1868–9–70.

	Years			Total
	1868	1869	1870	
Number of women attended in labour : natural .	511	443	442	1,396
" " " premature	4	1	15*	20
" " " married .	164	159	142	465
" " " single .	351	285	300	936
Males born	295	223	228	746
Females born	216	225	223	664
Mothers who died in or from labour . . .	2†	2‡	2§	6
Children born dead	79	58	58	195
Women confined at or above 40 years of age .	8	4	9	21
" " below 20 " .	105	98	81	284
Greatest age at delivery	46	42	44	—
Youngest "	17	16	15	—
Number of first confinements	223	207	105	535
Twin births	1	5	7	13
Triplets	0	0	1	1
Labours followed by flooding . . .	3	0	0	3
" accompanied by convulsions . . .	2	1	2	5
" " retained placenta . .	3	0	3	6
Forceps cases	7	4	4	15
Craniotomy cases	1	0	0	1
Version cases	2	0	1	3
Presentations : head	484	426	425	1,335
" breech	22	12	15	49
" feet	4	10	11	25
" arm	1	0	0	1

* Premature births : Seven months, 8; deaths, 5 : six months, 6; deaths, 6; five months, 1; death, 1.   † 1 puerperal convulsions, 1 bowel disease.
‡ 1 after instrumental labour, 1 metritis.   § 1 heart disease, 1 dropsy.

Subjoined is also a Table of the deaths and causes of death year by year for 13 years :—

Summary of Deaths and Causes of Death in the Lying-in Wards of Liverpool Workhouse for Years 1858–1870.

	1858	1859	1860	1861	1862	1863	1864	1865	1866	1867	1868	1869	1870
Morbus cordis . . .	2	—	1	—	—	1	—	—	—	—	—	—	1
Pneumonia . . .	1	—	—	—	—	1	—	—	—	1	—	—	—
Puerperal peritonitis .	1	1	—	1	6	—	2	2	3	—	—	—	—
Phthisis	1	—	—	—	1	—	1	—	—	1	—	—	—
Debility	2	—	—	—	—	—	—	—	—	—	—	—	—
Epileptic convulsions .	—	1	2	1	—	—	—	—	—	—	1	—	—
Puerperal fever . .	—	1	1	1	—	—	—	—	—	—	—	—	—
Jaundice . . .	—	1	—	—	—	—	—	—	—	—	—	—	—
Phlegmasia dolens .	—	1	—	—	—	—	—	—	—	—	—	—	—
Exhaustion . .	—	—	2	—	—	—	1	—	—	—	—	—	—
Relapsing fever .	—	—	1	—	—	—	—	—	—	—	—	—	—
Measles . . .	—	—	1	—	—	—	—	—	—	—	—	—	—
Inquest . . .	—	—	1	—	—	—	—	—	—	—	—	—	—
Laryngitis . . .	—	—	—	1	—	—	—	—	—	—	—	—	—
Obstructed labour .	—	—	—	1	—	—	—	—	—	—	—	—	—
Typhus, post partum .	—	—	—	1	—	—	—	—	—	—	—	—	—
Hæmorrhage . .	—	—	—	1	—	—	—	—	1	—	—	—	—
Uræmia . . .	—	—	—	—	—	1	—	—	—	—	—	—	—
Rupture of uterus .	—	—	—	—	—	—	—	1	—	—	—	—	—
Bright's disease .	—	—	—	—	—	—	—	—	—	1	—	—	—
Invaginated bowel .	—	—	—	—	—	—	—	—	—	—	1	—	—
Instrumental labour (fever)	—	—	—	—	—	—	—	—	—	—	—	1	—
Metritis . . .	—	—	—	—	—	—	—	—	—	—	—	1	—
Dropsy	—	—	—	—	—	—	—	—	—	—	—	—	1
Deaths	7	5	9	7	7	2	5	3	4	3	2	2	2
Approximate deliveries: * average estimated at 500 per ann.									450	625	511	443	442

* The approximate number of deliveries, 6396, given elsewhere, is rather under the mark than over, as will be seen by this Table, and is taken in order to be on the safe side. For, up to the three last years, the numbers are rather estimated than reckoned from the records. The total annual average deliveries calculated from different monthly records, i. e. 10 years of months = 500 in round numbers—1858–1867.

The three years 1868–9–70, for which only there are accurate records, speak for themselves ; and they show that the death-rate is marvellously low : not higher than in the healthy districts of England.

Let us now see what the arrangements are for this class of cases. The lying-in department of Liverpool workhouse is situated in a wing of the female general hospital, contiguous to the surgical wards. The wing has windows along the two opposite sides and at one end ; but the space is so divided off by partitions as to form five wards, each of which has windows along one side only. The wards are allotted in the following manner :—

Two of them, opening into each other, and facing the same way, contain each twelve double beds, affording accommodation for 24 inmates per ward, 48 in all, at 345 cubic feet per inmate. These two wards are devoted to the reception of pregnant women before delivery. The opposite half of the wing is divided into two wards, corresponding to the two pregnant wards ; one of these is the delivery ward, and contains seven beds, at nearly 1,200 cubic feet per bed.

Entering from this delivery ward is the lying-in ward, lighted by windows at the end. This ward contains 14 beds, at 900 cubic feet per bed. The other ward, entering from the delivery ward in the same line, is for convalescents, and contains eleven beds, at 762 cubic feet per bed. The W. C.'s, &c., are between the wards in the wing, in a very objectionable position.

For these and the following details I am indebted to the kindness of Mr. Barnes, who also supplied me with the statistics abstracted on Table V.

The following is the routine management of this establishment :—

All the wards are lime-washed three or four times a year. They are shut up and fumigated after the occurrence of any serious case of illness. The floors are washed daily.

The beds in the pregnant, lying-in, and convalescent wards,

are generally all or most of them occupied; but the number of occupied beds in the delivery ward rarely exceeds four or five.

The bed clothes are changed after each delivery, and the beds, which are of straw, after every third delivery.

The patients consist for the most part of unmarried women.[1] They are admitted into the pregnant wards, where they remain for a varying interval of from days to months, from whence they are removed to the delivery ward; about a fifth part of the women are admitted directly from the town to the delivery ward.

They remain on an average eight hours in the delivery room, whence they are removed to the lying-in ward, where they remain five or six days. They are then admitted to the convalescent ward, and are finally discharged fourteen days after labour, one half to the town, the other half into other parts of the workhouse.

An important part of the management is that the inmates of the pregnant wards only inhabit those wards at night, being engaged during the day in various occupations within the workhouse, but not about the lying-in women, as in the Paris Maternité.

Cases are not taken into the lying-in division unless labour has begun, or is supposed to be imminent.

Any case of illness occurring in the lying-in department is

---

[1] An attempt has been made in certain cases to account for the high death-rates of lying-in hospitals from the large proportion of unmarried women admitted. This opinion is directly contradicted by the experience of Liverpool workhouse, where out of 1,401 deliveries of women, 936 of whom, or two-thirds, were unmarried, there were only 6 deaths = 4·2 per 1,000 death-rate.

at once removed to the ' class sick nursery,' to the lock or other division.

The nurses engaged in the lying-in division attend also cases in the ' class sick nursery,' and are periodically changed. Any case which they cannot manage is referred to the resident medical officer on duty.

There are three of these officers, who relieve each other every eight hours day and night. The officer on duty is liable to be called on to visit any part of the workhouse or hospital during his turn of duty, so that it might happen occasionally that the medical officer might be called from the hospital to the lying-in division.

If feverish symptoms show themselves in any patient in the lying-in division, the practice is to isolate the case or to transfer it to some other division of the workhouse. The ward is then closed, fumigated, cleansed, and lime-washed, before being again used.

This proceeding has only been necessary twice within the last four years.

Until recently, the whole of the deliveries, which amounted to an average of about 500 a year, were under the charge of one paid officer and a pauper who, without any payment or extra diet, delivered nearly every case and worked both night and day.

There are several points in this procedure which are of great importance, as bearing on the general question of successful management of lying-in establishments :—

1. The building, although situated in a large commercial town, is on a high, isolated, and freely ventilated locality.

2. It is not connected with a general hospital or medical school, or with any of their risks.

3. There is a constant change of wards :—pregnant ward, delivery ward, lying-in ward, recovery ward, body of the house. There is, in short, as little risk as possible of the cumulative blood-poisoning process already referred to.

4. Frequent cleansing and lime-washing.

5. Passing women who have been delivered as speedily as possible out of the division altogether, either into the house or outside.

6. The deliveries being conducted by a woman specially attached to the delivery ward, and no part of whose duty it is to attend sick.

7. The immediate isolation or removal of all cases exhibiting feverish symptoms and their treatment out of the division.

8. The reduction of intercommunication between the lying-in and hospital divisions to the smallest possible degree on the part of medical officers and nurses.

The practical result of this system of management has been, as we have seen, that the lying-in division of this workhouse, although working under many singular disadvantages, has escaped the usual fatality of special lying-in hospitals.

During the thirteen years included in the tables there has been no epidemic, and the deaths have almost always been single and disconnected.

The experience of lying-in wards in London workhouses somewhat resembles the experience of Liverpool workhouse.

In the report of the committee appointed to consider the

cubic space of metropolitan workhouses, 1867, is given a table, No. 11, shewing the number of deliveries and deaths after delivery during five years in forty metropolitan workhouses.

The leading facts are abstracted in Table VI. Workhouses in which deaths after delivery took place, during the five years, are separated in the abstract from workhouses in which no deaths took place.

There were during these five years in all the workhouses 11,870 deliveries and 93 deaths, giving a death-rate of 7·8 per 1,000. The deaths from puerperal diseases amounted to 39, giving a death-rate of 3·3 per 1,000. There were 20 deaths from accidents of childbirth; being a death-rate of 1·7 per 1,000. The total death-rate due to both classes was 5 per 1,000.

The largest number of deliveries took place in Marylebone and in St. Pancras. In the former, on an average of 243 deliveries per annum, the death-rate was 8·2 per 1,000. One half of this, however, was due to consumption. Of the remaining deaths 3 were due to puerperal diseases (2·4 per 1,000) and 2 to accidents. The death-rate due to puerperal diseases and accidents of childbirth was thus 4·1 per 1,000.

In St. Pancras workhouse, on an average of 200 deliveries per annum, the death-rate was 11 per 1,000, of which 9 per 1,000 were due to puerperal diseases. Recent disclosures with regard to St. Pancras workhouse may to some extent account for this high death-rate. The number of deliveries in these two workhouses bring them almost within the category of lying-in hospitals.

There are four other workhouses in which the annual deliveries are respectively 171, 120, and two of them 111, while in all the others the numbers fall much below 100.

In one such instance (Holborn), where the deliveries have averaged fifty a year, the death-rate was exceptionally high, 24 per 1,000, one half of which was due to puerperal disease. In another instance, St. Mary's, Islington, with seventy-five deliveries per annum, the death-rate averaged 29 per 1,000. But the causes are not stated, and cannot now be ascertained. In Whitechapel, where there were 111 deliveries per annum, the death-rate was 10·8 per 1,000, one half being due to puerperal diseases.

It is possible that local enquiry might elucidate the causes of this mortality. The cases are, however, exceptional to the experience of London workhouses, viz. that the death-rates from puerperal diseases and accidents of childbirth are scarcely higher than they are in all England, town and country. Let us try to ascertain how far the management adopted may have led to these comparatively favourable results.

The conditions for recovery in a great majority of the London workhouse lying-in wards are at least as favourable as they are in the Liverpool workhouse; in most cases undoubtedly more so, as will immediately be seen when we consider that the average annual number of deliveries in Liverpool workhouse is more than twice that of the two largest London workhouses, and from five to ten times most of the others; that in the London workhouses the rule is to have many unoccupied beds, while this is the exception in the Liverpool workhouse.

The cardinal principle in the management of these London workhouse lying-in wards appears to be this : their occupants are a fluctuating number ; often the wards have but one woman at a time, and the cubic space for each of these women is ' in fact the cubic space of the whole ward.' [1] Sometimes, but only for brief periods, all the lying-in beds may be occupied. For much longer intervals the occupants are very few in number, so that each has a large proportion of cubic space, and sometimes the wards in some of the workhouses are empty. There are no medical schools attached to the institutions, and no medical students who may have passed from a case of erysipelas or from the post-mortem theatre to the lying-in bedside ; there is the possibility of removing immediately any case of febrile or other disease which may occur in the lying-in ward into the general sick wards of the workhouse ; there is discharge of convalescent cases at the earliest possible period, either to their own homes or to other parts of the establishment ; these conditions, together with the paucity of numbers and the occasional vacating and rest of the wards, appear to constitute the main difference between a workhouse lying-in ward and a lying-in hospital.

In both classes of establishments the same attention is doubtless bestowed on ventilation, cleanliness, and frequent change of bedding.

---

[1] In Lambeth and St. Pancras the wards are generally full.

MANAGEMENT OF MILITARY LYING-IN WARDS.

The lying-in arrangements provided for soldiers' wives are as follows :—

The rule is that women shall be delivered in quarters, provided there be decent accommodation. At a number of the larger stations, where suitable married quarters have not yet been fully provided, there are female hospitals, attached to which, as we have already seen, is a delivery and lying-in ward, with the usual offices. In the specially constructed hospitals the wards are of a good size, well-lighted, warmed and ventilated. If all the beds were occupied, the space would be 1,300 cubic feet per patient. But this is an event which rarely or never happens, so that there is always plenty of room and good ventilation.

If [1] a woman requires admission, her husband applies to the medical authorities for a ticket. No woman with a disease considered to be infectious is admitted. The women usually follow their ordinary avocations until obliged to proceed to hospital by imminent labour. They are taken there in cabs, all the necessary arrangements for the lying-in having been made, if possible, by previous inti-mation. The woman is delivered in the delivery ward, and is thence transferred to the lying-in ward. As a rule, the lying-in pavilion in these female hospitals is distinct in all its arrangements for nursing from the pavilion for general cases. Infectious cases are not received into the same hospital, except at Aldershot.

---

[1] These arrangements are commonly the same in civil lying-in institutions.

In these hospitals for soldiers' wives the time which elapses from the admission to the discharge of the women is usually ten, and in some cases twelve days.

At Aldershot four 'Sisters' are now at work in the soldiers' wives' hospital. One was trained as midwife, and took charge of the midwifery cases early in 1867. The Sister midwife has sole charge of the lying-in women for five or six days. They are then passed into a third ward, and are nursed by the Sisters who attend the ordinary cases (which are, however, of course in a separate ward).

The Sisters do not help the midwife, as a rule. Only the Superior, on an emergency, and one for scrubbing floors periodically, enter the midwifery wards (i.e. the delivery and lying-in wards).

In 1869 Aldershot had no fatal case among the lying-in women.

[The 'infection wards' are nursed by ordinary nurses, and in cases of children by the parents.]

It will be seen, therefore, that at Aldershot the midwife has nothing to do with the general cases, and the matron is not now the midwife. Both there and at Woolwich the lying-in nursing is quite separate from the general nursing.

The medical officer remarks, as to the two deaths in 1869 at Woolwich : 'Two cases of puerperal peritonitis after bad labours, requiring instrumental and other assistance, died, but the disease did not extend. My opinion is that the coldness of the wards, though objectionable, has a great deal to do with the comparative immunity hitherto enjoyed as regards the germination and extension of contagious diseases.'

It need scarcely be said that these new hospitals are models of cleanliness.

In the Colchester Hut the patient is received into a separate compartment, of which there are four, where she is delivered and remains until discharged to quarters.

It is very rarely indeed, if ever, that all the four compartments are occupied simultaneously. The average stay is ten days ; the average number of deliveries a year under 50.

This hut does not form part of a hospital. It is a separate establishment, solely for lying-in women, as such accommodation should always be.

Note.—There is another reason, though it may be termed a fanciful one, for altogether disconnecting lying-in institutions with general hospitals, and even with the name and idea of hospital. It is this : there must be a certain death-rate in a general hospital, receiving as it does fatal diseases and fatal accidents, as long as men and women have fatal diseases and fatal accidents.

But lying-in is not a fatal disease, nor a disease at all. It is not a fatal accident, nor an accident at all.

Unless from causes unconnected with the puerperal state, no woman ought to die in her lying-in ; and there ought, in a lying-in institution, to be no death-rate at all.

It is dangerously deadening our senses to this fact—viz., that there ought to be *no* deaths in a lying-in institution—if we connect it in the least degree with the name of hospital, so long as a hospital means a place for the reception of diseases and accidents.

In French statistics, this confusion of ideas, were it not

ghastly, would be ludicrous. 'Admissions,' under the head 'Malades,' include not only the lying-in women, but the new-born infants, which appear to be 'admitted' to life and to hospital together, as if life were synonymous with disease, so that, e.g. 4,000 'Admissions,' in such a year, to the Paris Maternité would mean 2,000 deliveries, 2,000 births— [and—how many deaths?]

RECAPITULATION.

In summing up the evidence regarding excessive mortality in lying-in institutions and its causes, it appears—

1. That, making every allowance for unavoidable inaccuracies in statistics of midwifery practice, there is sufficient evidence to show that in lying-in wards there reigns a death-rate many times the amount of that which takes place in home deliveries.

2. That a great cause of mortality in these establishments is 'blood-poisoning,' and that this arises from the greater susceptibility of lying-in women to diseases connected with this cause. From whence it follows that in many lying-in wards, as at present arranged and managed, there must be conditions and circumstances apart from those belonging to the inmates personally, which aid in the development of this morbid state.

3. That the risks to which lying-in women are exposed from puerperal diseases are increased by crowding cases in all stages into the same room or under the same roof; by retaining them for too long a period in the same room;

by using the same room for too long a period without cleansing, evacuation, rest, and thorough airing: but that the death-rate is not always in proportion to the number of lying-in cases which have passed through the hospital.

It follows from this that, other things being equal, a high death-rate may take place in a small hospital constantly used up to its capacity as well as in a large hospital constantly used up to its capacity.

4. That there are superadded causes in some establishments which add greatly to their dangers. Among these may be reckoned the following :—

(*a*) Prevalence of puerperal fever as an epidemic outside the hospital.

(*b*) Including midwifery wards within general hospitals, thereby incurring the risk of contaminating the air in midwifery wards with hospital emanations.

(*c*) Proximity to midwifery wards of post-mortem theatres or other external sources of putrescence.

(*d*) Admitting medical students from general hospitals or from anatomical schools to practice or even to visit in midwifery wards without special precautions for avoiding injury.

(*e*) Treating cases of puerperal disease in the same ward, or under the same roof, with midwifery cases.

(*f*) Permitting the same attendants to act in infirmary wards and in lying-in wards, and using the same bedding, clothing, utensils, &c., in both.

(*g*) Most probably also—especially in certain foreign hospitals—want of scrupulous attention to ventilation, and to cleanliness in wards, bedding, clothing, utensils, and patients, and in the clothing and personal habits of attendants.

In short, the entire result of this enquiry may be summed up, in a very few words, as follows :—A woman in ordinary health, and subject to the ordinary social conditions of her station, will not, if delivered at home, be exposed to any special disadvantages likely to diminish materially her chance of recovery. But this same woman, if received into an ordinary lying-in ward, together with others in the puerperal state, will from that very fact become subject to risks not necessarily incident to this state. These risks in lying-in institutions may no doubt be materially diminished by providing proper hospital accommodation, and by care, common sense, and good management. And hence the real practical question is, whether it is possible to ensure at all times the observance of these conditions.

The great mortality in lying-in hospitals everywhere is no doubt a strong argument against such a result being attainable ; so much so that, in the absence of this security, the evidence in the preceding pages appears sufficient to warrant the question being raised, whether lying-in hospitals, arranged and managed as they are at present, should not be forthwith closed ?

Can any supposed advantages to individual cases of destitution counterbalance the enormous destruction of human life shown by the statistics?

Without vouching for the entire accuracy of Le Fort's data, they may still be taken generally as showing approximately the penalty which is being paid for the supposed advantages of these institutions. It is this : (see Table XV.) for every two women who would die if delivered at home, fifteen must die if delivered in lying-in hospitals. Any reasonable deduction from this death-rate for supposed inaccuracy will not materially influence the result.

TABLE XV., *abstracted from* TABLES III. *and* X., *showing Comparative Mortality among Lying-in Women in Hospitals and at Home.*

	Deliveries	Deaths	Deaths per Thousand
Total for all hospitals . . .	888,312	30,394	34
Total delivered at home . . .	934,781	4,405	4·7
Excess of deaths per thousand delivered in hospitals			29·3

The evidence is entirely in favour of home delivery, and of making better provision in future for this arrangement among the destitute poor.

CAN THE ARRANGEMENT AND MANAGEMENT OF LYING-IN INSTITUTIONS BE IMPROVED ?

Must we, then, surrender the principle of lying-in institutions altogether, and limit the teaching of midwifery nurses solely to bedside cases at home, notwithstanding the well-known difficulties of teaching pupils at the beginning of their course elsewhere than in an institution ? We will try to reply to this question; and, in doing so, perhaps some

light may be thrown on another question, viz.: how to improve existing lying-in establishments so as to reduce the
mortality in them.

Evidence sufficient has been collected to show that no one
panacea will enable us either to possess a perfectly healthy
building, or to improve existing hospitals.

Much has been written about the saving effect of small
hospitals; but it is certain, from what has been already said,
that the small-hospital idea is not sufficient of itself. It is,
however, a very important idea, because all hospital prob-
lems are simplified by subdivision of the buildings. So far
as we know, every one who has carefully studied the subject
has given a preference to small lying-in establishments over
large ones; but we should certainly be disappointed if we
trusted to smallness of size alone for reducing the mortality.

The evidence further shows that in any new plan infirmary wards must be kept quite detached from lying-in
wards. They should be in another part of the ground, and
should be provided with their own furniture, bedding,
utensils, stores, kitchen, and attendants.

The same arrangement, at least in principle, should be
carried out at all existing lying-in establishments, and every
case of disease should at once be removed from the lying-in
wards to the infirmary, and be separately attended there.

In our proposed midwifery school the whole attendance
would be supplied by midwives and pupil midwives, with a
physician accoucheur, to make his visit twice a day, to be
sent for in time of need, and to give instruction to the pupil

midwives by lectures and otherwise; and in this way we should escape the dangers of introducing medical students.

Applying the same principle to lying-in wards to which medical students are admitted, there can be no doubt that a responsibility of the very gravest kind attaches to all teachers and managers of lying-in hospitals who do not satisfy themselves that students admitted as pupils have nothing to do, either with general hospital practice, or with anatomical schools, during the period. Midwifery instruction should be treated as a matter quite apart.

What has been already said need scarcely be repeated, about the dangers of connecting midwifery wards with general hospitals. The simple facts are sufficient to show that all midwifery wards of this class should be at once closed.

As a general result of this enquiry, applicable to all lying-in wards, the evidence shows that very much indeed of the success depends on good and intelligent administration and management.

Suppose that all these precautions could be carried out, will the cost and difficulty of giving effect to them necessarily lead to the abolition of all accommodation for midwifery cases, or for teaching midwifery?

We reply, No. The facts already adduced clearly show what may be done in this matter.

They prove, in the first place, that lying-in women should, as a rule, be delivered at home. And, as a consequence, that whatever provision may be made for cases of special destitution, or for midwifery teaching, such provision should be assimilated as far as practicable to the conditions which surround lying-in women in fairly comfortable homes.

These conditions are realised, and in some instances no doubt improved on, in the better class of workhouse lying-in wards, and of lying-in huts for soldiers' wives.

The favourable results arrived at in many of these institutions appear to show that a little more care would lower the death-rate still further.

In every instance where it is considered necessary to organise lying-in accommodation by voluntary effort, the same principles should be kept in view.

The success which has attended Waterford Lying-in Hospital, already mentioned, shows how much may be done in rendering such accommodation a real boon to the poor.

A single hut, like the Colchester Hut, erected in a needy locality, would supply, and that safely, all the accommodation wanted. But for a training school of midwives and midwifery nurses other accommodation is required, and of a far more costly character.

It is true that any sort of building may be leased or bought and altered, or added to, and told off as a training school; but after what has been said, to take such a course would be to ensure killing a certain number of mothers for the sake of training a certain number of midwives. If we are to have a training school at all, we must, before all things, make it as safe for lying-in women to enter it as to be delivered at home; and having made up our minds what is necessary for this purpose, we must pay for it.

CHAPTER II.

CONSTRUCTION AND MANAGEMENT OF A LYING-IN IN-
STITUTION AND TRAINING SCHOOL FOR MIDWIVES
AND MIDWIFERY NURSES.

To APPLY all this experience to the construction and
organisation of a school for midwives and midwifery
nurses[1] is the next thing :—

Everybody must be born, and every woman, at least in
this kingdom, is attended at the birth of her child by somebody, skilful or unskilful. Except in the case of multiple
births, there are therefore as many attendances as there
are births in the Returns of the Registrars-General.

This it is which makes the subject of midwifery nursing
of such paramount importance.

Lying-in is an operation which occurs in England to seven

---

[1] I call a midwife a woman who has received such a training, scientific and
practical, as that she can undertake all cases of parturition, normal and abnormal,
subject only to consultations, like any other accoucheur. Such a training could
not be given in less than two years.

I call a midwifery nurse a woman who has received such a training as will
enable her to undertake all normal cases of parturition, and to know when the
case is of that abnormal character that she must call in an accoucheur.

No training of six months could enable a woman to be more than a midwifery
nurse.

women out of a hundred annually. In 1868 there were 786,858 children born alive in this country, wherefore for the midwives and midwifery nurses to be trained there will always be occupation and custom enough ; whereas the occupation and custom for a surgical operator is, it is to be hoped, comparatively small, except in Franco-German wars. Even there we may trust that 7 out of 100 had not to undergo an operation. Certainly to 7 out of every 100 annually a surgical operation in England does not occur.

Between midwifery nursing and all other hospital nursing there is this distinction, viz. : the operator is herself the nurse ; and the head-operator (or midwife) ought to be a woman, and *is*, in Paris and Vienna, and elsewhere.

Lying-in patients are to be compared to surgical (or operation) patients, *not* to medical patients, and *should* be perfectly well in health.

Since lying-in is not an illness, and lying-in cases are not *sick* cases, it would be well, as already said, to get rid of the word ' hospital ' altogether, and never use the word in juxtaposition with lying-in women, as lying-in women should never be in juxtaposition with any infirmary cases.

As to amount of work, necessary administrative conveniences and the like, a lying-in institution is to be compared to a surgical, *not* medical hospital, or rather to a hospital for operations.

It has been already shown that great improvements are required in the manner of keeping midwifery statistics, and that many data are wanting for this purpose. It would be altogether wrong to deal with these statistics on the same principles as if they were general hospital statistics. Lying-in is neither a disease nor an accident, and any fatality attending it is not to be counted as so much per cent. of inevitable loss. On the contrary, a death in childbed is almost a subject for an inquest. It is nothing short of a calamity which it is right that we should know all about, to avoid it in future. A form of record is appended (Table XVI.), which appears to afford the means of registering the required information.

I. *CONSTRUCTION OF A LYING-IN INSTITUTION.*

What then, first, should be the principles of construction for a lying-in institution, in order to combine safety for the lying-in women with opportunity of training for the pupil midwives? And,

1. *How many Beds to a Ward?*

Not more than four.

Or single-bed wards might be arranged in groups of four.

Also, it must always be borne in mind that four beds mean eight patients. There are two patients to each bed (unless it is meant to kill the infants) to use up the air, which is besides used up by a necessarily far larger number of attendants than in any general hospital. For, during the time the mother is incapable of attending to the infant, the infant is incapable of attending to itself. Also, an exhausted

TABLE XVI.—*Proposed Registry of Midwifery Cases.*

Name	Age	Residence	Married or Single	No. of Pregnancy	Date when last Child was Born	Date of Admission	Period of Gestation	Date of Commencement of Labour	Duration of Labour, in hours	Nature of Delivery	Presentations	Complications of Delivery	Operation, if any	Nature of Accident or Disease	Date of Attack	Duration	Result and Date	Births : Single, Twins, or Triplets	Infant Born Living or Dead	Sex of Child	If Infant Dead after Birth, Cause of Death, and Date	Date of Removal from Lying-in Department	No. of Days in Lying-in Department	Date of Discharge from Institution	Remarks

NOTE.—Should any death take place in a woman discharged from the institution within a month from the time of her delivery, a record of this death, its date, and cause, to be entered in the column of Remarks. In the same column should be entered remarks on abnormal configuration, or on abnormal conditions of health which might influence the result of the delivery.

mother, and feeble, almost lifeless infant, cannot ring a bell or make themselves heard.   Indeed, an infant which cannot cry is in the greatest danger.

For all this provision must be made.   There are scarcely two points in common between a lying-in institution and a general hospital.

2. *How many Wards to a Floor?*

Only one four-bed ward, or four one-bed wards in a group.

3. *How many Floors to a Pavilion (hut or cottage)?*

Two, at most.   In every alternate pavilion better only one floor, unless the pavilions be so far apart as to cover an extent of ground which would make administration almost impossible, and cost fabulous.

How many Beds to a Pavilion or Hut?

There would therefore be no more than eight beds, and in each alternate pavilion no more than four beds.

How many Pavilions or Huts to a Lying-in Institution?

Not more than four two-floored pavilions, two one-floored pavilions, and two two-floored delivery pavilions; unless, indeed, building space can be given, with all its cost and administrative difficulties.

4. *How much space to the Bed?*

The *minimum* of ward cubic space for a lying-in woman, even where the delivery ward is, as it ought always to be, separate, is 2,300 cubic feet in a single-bed ward, and 1,900 cubic feet in a four-bed ward.

[In ordinary army wooden huts, where the air comes in at every seam, this space may be less.]

As it is a principle that superficial area signifies more than cubic space, the surface of floor for each bed should not be less than 150 square feet per bed in a four-bed ward, and in a single-bed ward not less than 190 square feet, because this is the total available space for all purposes in a single-bed ward. This space has to be occupied, not only by the lying-in woman and her infant, and perhaps a pupil midwife washing and dressing it at the fire, but often by the midwife, an assistant, possibly the medical officer, and pupil midwives. In a four-bed ward there is space common to all the beds.

The Delivery Ward

Ought to be separate in every lying-in institution; *must* be separate in an institution of more than four or five beds, though in separate compartments.

Every delivery bed should have a superficial area of not less than 200 square feet, and a cubic space of not less than 2,400 cubic feet.

5. *How many Windows to a Bed?*

One at least to each bed. Two beds and two windows on each side of the four-bed ward.

In a single-bed ward the bed should not be placed directly between window and door. And it must never be in an angle. There must be room for attendants on both sides the bed.

This is still more essential in a delivery ward. Each bed should be lighted on *both* sides by windows, and should have at least five feet of passage room on either side.

6. *What are healthy Walls and Ceilings and Floors?*

Oak floors, polished; furniture also; impervious glazed walls and ceilings, or frequent lime-washing.

All that has been so justly said as to the necessity of impervious polished floors and walls for hospitals applies tenfold to lying-in institutions, where the decomposition of dead organic matter, and the re-composition of new organic matter, must be constantly going on.

It is this, in fact, which makes lying-in institutions so dangerous to the inmates.

And it may literally be said that the danger increases as the square of the number of in-cases.

Lying-in ' infection ' is a very good illustration of what ' infection ' really means, since *parturition* is not infectious or ' contagious.'

The excessive susceptibility of lying-in women to poisonous emanations, the excessively poisonous emanations from lying-in women—these constitute a hospital influence on lying-in cases brought together in institutions, second to no influence we know of exercised by the most 'infectious' or 'contagious' disease.

The death-rate is not much higher among women lying-in at home in large towns than in healthy districts. Therefore the agglomeration of cases together and want of management required to meet it must bear the blame.

As to floors, the well-laid polished floor is *a sine quâ non* in a lying-in institution, where, with every care, slops, blood, and the like, must frequently be spilt on the floor.

7. *What is a healthy and well-lighted Delivery Ward?*

There must be two separate delivery wards for each floor of the whole lying-in institution, so arranged and connected *under cover* that the lying-in women may be removed after delivery to their own ward. And for this purpose the corridors must admit of being warmed during winter, especially at night, so as to be of a tolerably equable temperature.

Unlimited hot and cold water laid on, day and night, W.C. sink, bath-sink, clean linen, must be close at hand.

In a pavilion hospital one single-bed ward should be attached to each delivery ward, for an exhausted case after delivery, till she is able to be moved to her own ward.

The delivery ward should be so lighted and arranged that it can be divided, by curtains only, into three if not four compartments.

No woman being delivered should see another delivery going on at the same time.

The delivery bedsteads stand in their compartments.

Each delivery bed should have window light on either side, and also ample passage room all round and on both sides the bed.

Care should be taken that no bed should stand exactly between door and window, on account of draughts.

The curtains, of washing material, are only just high enough to exclude sight, not high enough to exclude light or air, and are made so as to pull entirely back when not wanted. Each area enclosed by the curtains should of course be sufficiently ample for pupils, attendants, and patient; also for a low truck on broad wheels covered with india-rubber, to be brought in, on which the bedstead with the clean warm bedclothes is placed, and the newly delivered woman conveyed to her own ward.

[A woman very much exhausted would be carried in the delivery bed to the bye-ward attached to each delivery ward.]

The reason why there must be two delivery wards for each floor of a lying-in institution, to be used alternately, one 'off,' one 'on,' is that one delivery ward on each floor must be always vacant for thorough cleansing, lime-washing and rest for a given period, say month and month about.

It is understood that newly-delivered women cannot be removed from one floor to another. And it is quite necessary to have the means of keeping a corridor, along which a newly-delivered woman is to be moved, at a proper temperature.

The position of the delivery wards should be as nearly as possible equidistant from the lying-in wards, and should be such that the women in labour, on their way to the delivery ward, need not to pass the doors of other wards.

A separate scullery to each delivery ward is indispensable; such scullery to be on at least an equal scale to that of ward sculleries. Hot and cold water to be constantly at hand, night and day. A sink-bath is desirable for immediately putting in water soiled linen from the beds and the like.

The scullery should contain a linen-press, small range with oven, hot closet at side of the fire-place, sink with hot and cold water, &c. A small compartment should contain a slop sink for emptying and cleansing bed-pans, and a sink about six inches deep and sunk below the floor, which is intended for filling and emptying a portable bath, and which when not required for this might be used for soaking linen, &c.

Beyond the scullery, so as to be as far removed as may be from the traffic of the main corridor and the noises of the delivery ward, should be the bye-ward, with not less than 2,100 cubic feet of contents.

8. Scullery, Lavatory, W.C.

The necessary consumption of hot and cold water is at least double or triple that of any general hospital. Sinks and W.C. sinks must be everywhere conveniently situated.

There must be a scullery to each four beds; the scullery

G

must needs be much larger and more convenient than in a
general hospital. There is often more work to be done by
night than by day in a lying-in institution.

All the ward appurtenances, scullery, lavatory, &c., must
stand empty for thorough cleansing, when the ward to
which they belong stands empty in rotation for this purpose,
and must not be used for any other ward. For each four-
bed ward, or group of four one-bed wards, or for each floor
of each pavilion, there must therefore be one scullery, with
a plentiful unfailing supply of hot and cold water, with sinks
and every convenience. The reason for this is two-fold :—

(1) To allow each scullery, with the other ward offices, to
be thoroughly cleansed and whitewashed with its own
group of four beds.

(2) The work in a scullery and in all the other ward
appurtenances day and night, night and day, is many-fold
that which it is in a general hospital scullery.

Besides this, general hospital patients ought never to be
allowed to enter the scullery.

In a lying-in scullery the infants, most exacting of all
patients, must frequently be in the scullery.

Even under the very best circumstances there are
many lying-in cases among weakly women where the
mother's state is such as to render it necessary for a ' cry-
ing ' infant to be washed and dressed elsewhere than in its
mother's ward. These infants are best washed, in that case,
in the scullery, which must be so arranged that infants
can be washed and dressed without being exposed to a
thorough draught, and that nurses and babies may not be
hustling one another.

There must be a good press in each scullery. A supply of clean linen and other necessaries will have to be kept in each press in each scullery.

The slop-sink and other appurtenances must be arranged so as to make allowance for the fact that the going backwards and forwards for water, hot and cold, or to empty slops in a lying-in institution—where half the patients can do nothing for themselves, and the other half (the mothers) are supposed to be ready for discharge when they can go to the ward offices for themselves—is more than it is in general hospitals.

Fixed baths are not necessary. But there must be means for filling with hot water moveable infants' baths at all hours at a moment's notice, since an infant's life often depends on immediate facility of hot-water bathing.

And this besides the daily regular night and morning washing of infants.

There must be also a moveable bath for each ward for the lying-in women, with the means for supplying it with hot and cold water and for emptying it. Lying-in patients are not able to use either fixed baths or lavatory.

Glazed earthenware sinks should alone be used, as being by far the safest and cleanest.

9. *How to Ventilate Lying-in Wards.*

The best ventilation is from opposite windows. Each window should be in three parts, the third or uppermost to consist of a flap hung on hinges to open inwards and throw the air from without upwards.

Inlet valves, to admit fresh air, and outlet shafts, to emit foul air, must be added to complete the natural ventilation.

10. *Furniture, Bedding, Linen.*

As little ward furniture as possible. As much clean linen as possible.

A very large and convenient clean linen-store, light and dry, must be assigned to the matron : very much larger than would be required for a general hospital ; but no general hospital in London supplies a good standard for such.

There must be in each scullery, besides, a clean linen-press.

There should be a very ample and convenient place for bedding.

Mattresses, blankets and the like, have to be renewed, taken to pieces and washed—especially those used in the delivery ward—many times oftener than in any general hospital.

The rack for linen should be along the middle of the linen-store.

There should be space for a bedding-rack along one end, taking about three feet six inches from the length of the room for linen. Space for some spare mattresses and bolsters will be necessary ; and they should be stowed near to a lift.

A linen-store requires thorough lighting, ventilating, and warming. Three windows are better than one. The linen must of course be kept dry and aired.

11. *Water Supply, Drainage, Washing.*

Unlimited hot and cold water supply, day and night, should be laid on all over the buildings.

All drains and sewers must be kept outside the walls of the buildings, and great care should be bestowed on trapping and ventilating them, to prevent foul air passing into the institution.

The washing in a lying-in institution is, it need not be said, very large, and should be conducted quite at a distance. Sink-baths, for immediately putting in water soiled-linen, are necessary.

12. *Medical Officer's Room and Waiting-room.*

No dispensary, especially no dispenser, is needed in a lying-in institution.

A medical officer's room is necessary. The medical officer is not resident. He makes his morning and evening visit, and is called in by the head midwife for any difficult case. He gives instruction, scientific and practical, to the pupil midwives. [These lectures are given in the pupil midwives' mess-room.]

In the medical officer's room should be kept the instruments, to which a fully qualified head midwife also has a key. The medical officer keeps the notes of cases, &c., and of instruction to the pupil midwives in this room.

The few, very few, drugs needed in a good lying-in institution are kept here, or in the head midwife's sitting-room.

A waiting-room is necessary.

There must be a room where the head midwife can examine a woman, to know if labour is imminent.

This might be done in the medical officer's room or the waiting-room.

13. *Segregation Ward.*

A ward is unfortunately necessary, completely isolated, where a sick case, brought in with small-pox or erysipelas or the like, could be delivered and entirely separated from the others, or where a case of puerperal fever or peritonitis (though such ought never to arise after delivery in a properly constructed and managed institution) could be transferred. But if, unfortunately, puerperal fever should appear in the hospital, no new admissions should be allowed until the buildings have been thoroughly cleansed, lime-washed, and aired.

The segregation ward must have a nurse's room, and a provision of sink, slop-sink, &c.

14. *Kitchen.*

The kitchen should be well placed, conveniently near, yet sufficiently cut off from the main corridor by a neck of passage and intermediate offices.

SITE.

The site of a lying-in institution must be open, airy, surrounded with its own grounds, not adjoining or near to any other building, still less to any hospital or any nuisance or source of miasm. But it must be in the immediate vicinity of any large centre of population from which the lying-in women come.

And this involves the question of receiving-rooms.

Should there be a receiving-room, as well as a waiting-room?

The lying-in woman's name is put down for admission some time beforehand.

Lying-in hospitals differ as to their rules whether or no to admit women any time before labour is imminent. If they are not so admitted, they often have to be sent back again home.

It is now believed to be the soundest principle that the fewer days a lying-in woman spends in a lying-in institution, beyond the time she is actually under treatment, the better; and this involves that she should not be admitted till labour is imminent—even at the risk of the infant being born in cab or lift (which *has* happened).

Lying-in institutions must (unfortunately) be, therefore, in the immediate neighbourhood of great towns or centres of population.

[Even those London Boards which are building their excellent new workhouse infirmaries in the country, are forced to keep their lying-in wards in the old workhouses in the town.]

The difference, however, as has been shown by our statistics, is not so great between the mortality of women lying-in at home in the country and in the town as should make us pronounce against lying-in institutions in great centres of population—provided they have a large and entirely isolated area completely to themselves, perhaps a proportion of two acres to fifty beds.

But this involves another question.

A large proportion, alas! of workhouse lying-in women (we have seen two-thirds at Liverpool [1]) are unmarried. Of these many have no home.

It is difficult to send these women back again, even if labour is not actually imminent. And it is impossible to send them out after delivery, till recovery is fairly confirmed.

In workhouses the question is solved by women being admitted into the body of the house during pregnancy, and discharged into the body of the house, if not to their own homes, when quite convalescent.

In Liverpool Workhouse fourteen days after labour the lying-in women are thus discharged. Fourteen, eighteen, twenty-one days, are the average of a woman's stay in the lying-in division in London workhouses.

A soldiers' wives' hospital takes in no unmarried women to lie-in.

Civil lying-in institutions almost invariably have to make exceptions and take in unmarried women.

In workhouses they are not the exception, they are the rule. Married women are the exception.

It is to be observed that married women will rarely come in an hour before, or stay an hour after it is necessary, in any lying-in institution.

Ten to twelve days is 'the average period of hospital

---

[1] In some London workhouses it is yet larger.

treatment' in Colchester, Woolwich, and other soldiers' wives' lying-in hospitals. 'Women of this station of life cannot, as a rule, be prevailed upon to submit to longer detention,' it is added.

The average number of days in King's College Hospital lying-in ward was sixteen. None were permitted to leave under fourteen days. Twenty-one days were *allowed*, in ordinary cases. It is feared this might be too long; but so very many weakly, half-starved women sought admission, that to send some away sooner was 'to ensure a break-down,' it is stated.

In a civil lying-in institution it would not be by any means desirable absolutely to exclude single young women *primiparæ*; it would be grievous to some of these poor things to be sent among the (often hardened) wretched women of the workhouse. The whole question of these poor young women—unmarried mothers of a first child—is full of difficulty. It would never do, morally, to make special provision for them. And for this very reason we seem bound to receive such, conditionally, into well regulated lying-in institutions, and afford some kindly care to prevent, at the very least, their sinking lower. But it would not be right to leave any admissions for single women in the hands of any young assistant, or morally inexperienced person.

The principle appears to be that, if pregnant women are to be received some time before and kept some time after delivery, the excess of time should not be passed in the lying-in wards, but in separate accommodation.

II. *MANAGEMENT*.

Construction, however, in a lying-in institution, holds only the second place to good management in determining whether the lying-in patients shall live or die. And without such management, no construction, however perfect, will avail.

And the first elementary principle of good management is to have always one pavilion of four or eight beds, according as it is of one floor or of two, standing empty in rotation for purposes of thorough cleansing. *A fortiori*—one delivery pavilion on each floor is always to be vacant alternately.

The pavilion to be in rotation unoccupied for the purposes of cleansing must necessarily be the *whole* pavilion, with all its sculleries and ward offices, since the process of cleansing is—turning out all the little furniture a lying-in ward ought ever to possess, bringing in lime-washers, possibly scrapers and painters, leaving doors and windows open all day, and even all night.

Every reason for having each ordinary pavilion ward completely separate, and individually *pavilionised*, applies with tenfold force to the delivery ward. Each must be complete in itself, with all its appurtenances and bye-ward for extreme cases, as a little pavilion. There is no possibility for properly cleansing and lime-washing the delivery ward *not* in use, unless this be the case.

One delivery ward, however spacious and well arranged

constantly used, would be a centre of deplorable mischief for the whole institution. This makes *two* delivery wards for each floor of the institution indispensable, to be used alternately for the whole floor at given periods.

N.B. Liverpool Workhouse with 25 lying-in beds, exclusive of delivery beds, has had an average of 500 deliveries *a year* for eleven years. A civil lying-in hospital in or near a large town is generally *just as full as it is permitted* to be. Five or six hundred deliveries or more *a year* might be reckoned upon; occasionally three or four deliveries a night. Sculleries will be *always* in use, *day and night*. All this renders it imperative that an inexorable rule should be made and kept to, viz. that every lying-in pavilion should be vacant in rotation, each delivery pavilion alternately, for thorough cleansing.

2. The second elementary principle of good management is to remove every case of *illness* arising in the institution, and every such case admitted into the institution, at once to an isolated sick ward or infirmary ward.

This is *must*, not may.

Though we should have no puerperal fever or peritonitis in a building of this *make*, yet unfortunately other institutions will send in (say) erysipelas or small-pox patients seized with labour.

Sad experience tells that this unprincipled practice has often proved fatal to many other inmates of the lying-in institution, turning an institution into a hospital.

Every sick case should therefore be completely isolated, in a separate sick ward, from the lying-in women. And if admitted before delivery, her delivery should take place in this separate ward.

N.B. The nurse's dinner and meals may be prepared in the general kitchen and sent to her. The patient's arrow-root, gruel, &c., must be made, and her beef-tea warmed, in the 'sick or segregation' building, and all linen must be sent to the ward well aired.

Is it desirable to connect the 'segregation' ward by any covered passage with the rest of the lying-in institution?

There is much to be said for and against.

The ward, it is to be hoped, will not often have to be used at all.

But small-pox has appeared after labour.

There might be danger in taking a patient from the institution to this ward through the open air, in all weathers, unprotected by any covered passage.

On the other hand, when once the patient is in the ward, complete isolation is by far the best, for the sake of all the others.

And there is by no means the same necessity for a passage as in the other parts of the institution where any night there may be three or four ordinary delivery cases to be conveyed through the passages.

A covered ambulance for sick cases is not, however, a nice thing, though often suggested.[1]

---

[1] The only difficulty is as to protecting the patient (a lying-in woman) during the transit in cold or wet weather; but perhaps some cover might be contrived for the bed or litter on which she is carried, which would be light, easily removable, and which could be exposed to the free action of the open air when not in use.

3. The first two may be called universal and essential principles of good management in every lying-in institution, large or small, however perfectly constructed.

Here is a third, hardly less essential, wherever there is more than one bed to a ward, viz. to remove a lying-in woman three times during her stay in the institution.

The average course of an ordinary case may be reckoned thus:—

Seven or eight hours in the delivery ward.

Five or six days in the lying-in ward.

Nine or ten days in the convalescent ward.

The nearer wards to the delivery ward in use should always be made the wards for women immediately after delivery; the farther wards for the same women when removed for their convalescent stage.

In a single-bed ward the woman may remain in her own ward from after her delivery till her discharge ; that is, no further removal after her delivery is necessary.

4. Cases of extreme exhaustion after delivery, which are better out of the delivery ward yet cannot be moved many yards, should be carried *in their beds* to the bye-ward adjoining the delivery ward, till they are somewhat recovered.

These must have a constant watcher by them.

5. In a lying-in institution about three times the quantity of linen and bedding for each patient is necessary of what is used at a general hospital.

The day's and night's provision of linen is kept in each ward scullery, and in the scullery of each delivery ward in use.

The linen-store in the store-room, and the bedding-store, need to be very complete and ample.

The bedding, that is, the mattress and blankets, of any one bed in the delivery ward should not be used for more than three or four delivery cases in succession without undergoing some process of purification—and this quite independent of any accident, the mattress of course being protected by Macintosh sheeting.

III. TRAINING SCHOOL FOR MIDWIVES.

The few words which will here be added on the management of a midwifery training school are not at all to be understood as a manual for practical instruction, which it is quite impossible to introduce here, but as simply treating of the management, in so far as this determines some constructive arrangements as imperative, and others as to be avoided.

No charity or institution, I believe, could possibly bear the expense of a single-bed ward, or even of a four-bed ward lying-in establishment, for a pretty constant succession of thirty-two patients, unless there were a training school.

[Thirty-two single-bed wards, an administrator would say, would require sixteen nurses, independently of midwives!!]

Even with a training school, the first year would be one of great difficulty, since all well managed training schools 'take in' pupils as much as possible at only two periods of the year, so as never to have the whole of the pupils fresh hands at once. But the *first* batch must necessarily be all fresh hands. A raw girl cannot be turned in to sit up with a newly-delivered woman and new-born infant. And a midwife cannot be spared to each girl all to herself, to teach her how to handle an infant. [That is, in each single-bed ward.]

The whole nursing service of a large four-bed or one-bed ward lying-in institution is so complicated, so different from that of a general hospital with its 20 or 32-bed wards, that it is difficult to provide for.

In even guessing at what the nursing accommodation should be for so completely new an experiment as a lying-in institution of 40 beds in single-bed or four-bed pavilions, we must begin by stating the probable requirements, the whole being tentative.

The staff would have to be at least as follows :—

One matron.

One head midwife.

One assistant midwife.

One deputy assistant midwife (for the first year).

To establish a really good training school,

Thirty pupil midwives.

[Two experienced good nurses in addition might be necessary for the first year.]

One cook.

One housemaid.

One or two other female servants, such as scourers—or more (number required depending on the flooring used).

Though this staff appears enormous, it is calculated upon the plan of giving only one night nurse to every four beds, —upon the supposition that 32 occupied beds will give a constant succession of cases, enough to provide instruction for almost as many pupil midwives ;—upon the principle that for systematic instruction there must be a fair number of pupils ; as, if every moment of their time is occupied in active duties, they cannot be well trained ;—and also upon the obvious fact that it would be impossible, from its extravagance, to nurse such a construction without pupils.

[For the *second* year, if a portion of the pupils are to be made thorough midwives, and their time of training two years, possibly the deputy-assistant midwife, and probably both the nurses, might be dispensed with.

The second-year pupil midwives ought to be quite competent, each to be in charge of two or three first-year's pupils and several patients, taking these patients from the beginning, and teaching pupils to handle new-born infants, look after ordinary lying-in cases, and the like ; and most excellent practice it is for the young teachers.]

As to scourers, the nature of the floors decided upon will determine what are wanted.

Also, none of the midwives can be expected to be housemaids, even in their own rooms. They have too much to do. The pupil midwives would be expected to clean their own bed-rooms, but not to scour, either for the patients or for themselves.

There must be a common room for pupil midwives. Here they take their meals in detachments. Head midwife, as a rule, with first detachment ; matron carving. Here they receive lectures and instruction from the physician accoucheur.

The matron must have two rooms.

The head midwife may have two rooms. She will expect to have her tea in her own room.

The head midwife, her assistants, and all her staff, should be lodged in a central position, and there should be ready means of communication with these quarters, both by bells and speaking tubes, from each pavilion and delivery ward.

A regular night service in a lying-in institution being impossible, the head midwife, when she goes her last round at night, say between eleven and twelve P.M., stations other watchers for any emergency arising besides those now to be mentioned, who are for the night nursing of ordinary cases.

For this one pupil would probably be told off for each four wards or beds, and one extra for the whole floor, who must not be an inexperienced pupil. Her duty would be to visit each pavilion on her floor, and to have all in readiness in the delivery ward for cases coming in at night—a not infrequent occurrence.

The head midwife would also arrange for the special care of any critical case at once, on the patient being conveyed to her own ward, or to that adjacent to the delivery ward.

In so large and therefore busy a lying-in institution, it would not be desirable to call up all the pupil midwives to every case coming in the night. They would be appointed day by day alternately, and the number told off for the purpose would be called to any case coming *that* night.

It is therefore most desirable that the sleeping-rooms or compartments (each with its own window) of the pupil midwives should be arranged in at least three reliefs, so that the occupants of one dormitory, or relief, could be called by a bell from the delivery ward ringing into that dormitory without needlessly disturbing others.

In so large an institution the head midwife even cannot attend every night case.

The assistant must be a well qualified midwife, who can take her turn in attending night cases, calling the head midwife if necessary.

Through all this organization, however, as far as possible, each pupil is told off to be in charge of a mother and infant from beginning to end.

And there will always be unfortunately a certain number of cases, each requiring a nurse constantly by her side day and night.

It is obvious that the same woman cannot do this for a succession of days and nights.

But the number of severe cases requiring it would unquestionably be much smaller in a single-bed ward hospital, or in a four-bed ward hut hospital, because of its superior immunity from puerperal disease ; though, from the single-bed ward condition, every such case will require a nurse all to itself. And the same nurse cannot be always sitting up day and night.

N.B. Repetitions may possibly here be pardoned. The pupil midwife appointed as night watcher for the whole floor cannot be depended upon to attend the bell of any individual watcher. She may be absent at a delivery.

Yet the life of an infant, *e.g.*, in convulsions, depends on minutes—on the watcher being able to summon immediate help, hot water for a bath, and the like.

Those appointed to be called in such emergency should therefore be readily communicated with by bells or otherwise, without disturbing others, either nurses or patients.

As there are no sleeping-rooms for any midwife or pupil in the ward pavilions, it is necessary to insist upon this—that there should be every facility for their being rung up or called up at night.

Every pupil midwife ought to have a little bedroom to herself, or at least a compartment with half a window, or better a whole window, to itself. There should be a bathroom and W.C. on each floor in the pupil nurses' quarters, and a back staircase.

If a small sick-room could be managed for pupil midwives, it would be advisable. Where there are so many, one may be attacked with bronchitis or with scarlatina. She could not, of course, be 'warded' with the lying-in women; and it might be undesirable to leave her in her own little room, though this is quite sufficient for any slight illness. The top floor, as securing greater quiet, and a certain degree of isolation, might be the best for this sick-room.

The whole of the pupil midwives' quarters should have direct and ready means of communication with the hospital proper. Each relief should be independent of the other two, and under the immediate supervision of the official woman, whose quarters are attached to its own.

It need scarcely be stated that an essential part of a Pupil Midwife's training is to attend lying-in women at their own homes, with the conveniences or rather the inconveniences

of those homes. Otherwise the Pupil will be the less fit for
her after-work. The last two months of every six might
well be given to this. But, as above said, these 'Notes'
about management, for they are nothing more, simply treat
of it as regards construction, and do not refer to the necessary training, either in-door or out-door, at all.[1]

DESCRIPTION OF SKETCH-PLANS OF PROPOSED
INSTITUTION.

I know of no single building which requires more in-
genuity to plan, and has hitherto received less, than a lying-
in institution, especially with a training school for midwives
attached.

Lieut. Ommanney, R.E., has been kind enough to give
his time and mind to the subject—having previously had
considerable experience at the War Office in planning female
hospitals—and to embody the whole of the working accommodation required for both lying-in institution and school in the
thoughtfully arranged sketch-plans, Nos. III., IV., and V.

The estimated cost of these plans is large; but if we must
have lying-in institutions at all, it is only 'penny wise and
pound foolish' to cripple either space or necessary appliances, or the means of regularly and periodically vacating
every ward and every ward-office destined for the use of
lying-in women.

---

[1] For a great part of the foregoing details of management I am indebted to
the valuable experience of her, who, as then Superior of the nursing at King's
College Hospital, conducted our Training School for Midwifery Nurses there, so
kindly, so wisely, and so well, that its necessary breaking up was the more to
be deplored by all.

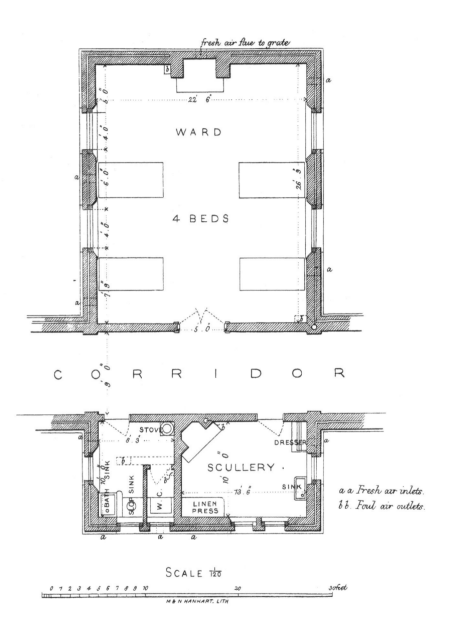

fresh air flue to grate

WARD

4 BEDS

22' 6"

26' 9"

5. 0

C O R R I D O R

9' 0"

STOVE

DRESSER

SCULLERY .

BATH

SINK

SINK

W.C.

LINEN PRESS

SINK

8.3

13. 6"

10' 0"

a a Fresh air inlets.
b b Foul air outlets.

S C A L E 1/120

0 1 2 3 4 5 6 7 8 9 10   20   30 feet

M & N HANHART. LITH

W. F. OMMANNEY.
LT. R.E

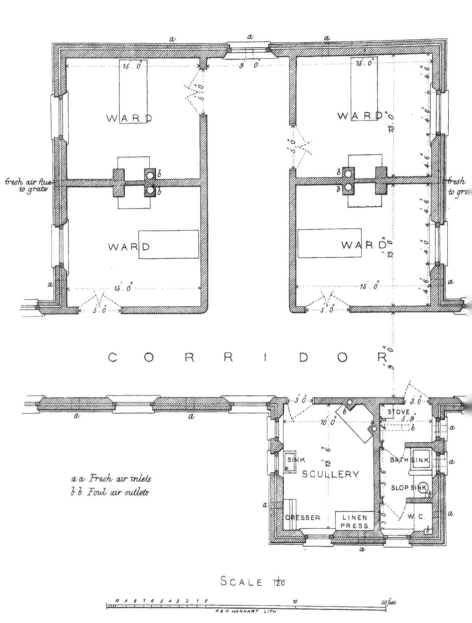

a.a Fresh air inlets
b.b. Foul air outlets

SCALE ⅟₁₂₀

W. F OMMANNEY
Lᵀ R.E.

PLAN III.

This plan shows a lying-in ward unit for the institution, together with its scullery and separate offices, and the relation which these bear to the corridor of communication joining all parts of the hospital on each floor together.

The measurements and other details shown on this plan are the result of repeated and careful consideration of the requirements already described; and it is believed that in practice they would be found sufficient for every purpose.

The four beds shown on it are not the *minimum*, but the *maximum* number which, judging from all past experience, could be safely placed together.

PLAN IV.

Shows a floor of one of the lying-in ward pavilions, divided into four separate one-bed rooms. This plan also represents a unit, but of another construction. The great advantage of the arrangement is complete separation of cases from each other, so that each room is as far as possible assimilated to a room in a private dwelling-house. To obtain this advantage the rooms are arranged in pairs on each side of a nine-feet passage, having a window at one end and a corridor-window opposite the other end.

Two of the rooms open from the corridor, and two rooms from the passage, but the doors are not opposite each other. In this, as in the four-bed ward plan, the scullery and offices are completely isolated from the rooms by a nine-feet corridor. In this case, also, the measurements and other details have been arrived at after full consideration. This plan would be somewhat more costly than the previous one (Plan III.). The justification of it is found in the fact that it reproduces, in a permanent form, the conditions in Colchester Lying-in Hut, already described. And in this hut there has, as yet, been no death after delivery.

PLAN V.

A lying-in institution for forty beds (thirty-two to thirty-six occupied), with a training school for thirty pupil midwives and midwifery nurses.

This plan gives a sketch of an arrangement of pavilions, offices, quarters, &c., forming a complete lying-in institution and training school. As already stated, such an institutiom must, from its very objects, be situated in a town where land is scarce and valuable, and this is a chief difficulty in erecting it. Hence it has been necessary to keep the different parts as close together as possible, and yet not to crowd them so as to interfere injuriously with the external ventilation. The mere architecture, as will be seen, has been subordinated to this necessity, but it must be borne in mind that utility, and not architectural effect, is to be sought for.

In the centre of the plan project the quarters for pupils, on three floors, ten quarters on each floor. They are arranged in this way to enable the reliefs to be taken from one floor at a time. Behind these, in the same block, are quarters for matron and midwives, waiting-room, surgery, stores, kitchen, and pupils' dining-room. The general entrance is in one side of the centre block. The two front pavilions, on either side the centre, contain the delivery wards, two on each floor. Each delivery pavilion contains a ward for three beds on each floor, with its bye-ward and offices. Only one delivery pavilion will be in use at one time. While one pavilion is in use, the other will be vacant, and undergoing ventilation and cleansing. These delivery-wards are connected with the centre, and with all the pavilions on each floor by a nine-feet corridor, with cross-light and ventilation. Fire-places are shown for warming in winter. On the ground-floor are three four-bed wards, with offices, on each side, on the construction shown on Plan III. There will thus be twenty-four lying-in beds, and six delivery beds (but three delivery beds and 20 lying-in beds only in use at the same time) on the ground floor. The second pavilion from the front, on each side, is only one storey in height, so as to afford a freer circulation of air among the pavilions in the space within which it might be necessary to place them.

As a consequence of this arrangement there would be only four lying-in wards, of four beds each, on the upper floor, together with a delivery ward at each side (one delivery ward to be used at a time).

A special detached ward for febrile cases is shown behind the building.

The total accommodation in an establishment of this size would be sufficient for 6 simultaneous deliveries and 32 to 36 lying-in women. There would be 6 delivery beds always resting, and 4 or 8 lying-in beds always unoccupied. There would be training accommodation and facilities for 30 pupils.

PLAN V

PLAN
OF A
LYING IN INSTITUTION.
FOR 40 (32 TO 36 OCCUPIED) BEDS
With Training School for 30 Pupil Midwives.

REFERENCE

A   Administration.
B   Kitchen and Stores.
C   Delivery Pavilions.
D   Ward Pavilions.
E   Segregation Pavilion.

note. The parts diagonally shaded
are one story only in height.

GROUND FLOOR PLAN

FIRST FLOOR PLAN

SECOND FLOOR PLAN

The material originally positioned here is too large for reproduction in this reissue. A PDF can be downloaded from the web address given on page iv of this book, by clicking on 'Resources Available'.

APPENDIX.

MIDWIFERY AS A CAREER FOR EDUCATED WOMEN.

My dear Sisters (or rather, Chers et très-honorés Confrères),

While all that we women think about is to have the same education as men in medicine, must we not feel the women's medical movement to be rather barren when it might be so fruitful?

But public opinion in England is not free enough for a coward to dare to say what she thinks, unless at the risk of having her head (figuratively) broken.

Is there not a much better thing for women than to be 'medical men,' and that is to be *medical women*?

Has not the cart been put before the horse in this women's medical movement?

Here is a branch so entirely their own, that we may safely say that no lying-in would be attended but by a woman if a woman were as skilful as a man—a physician accoucheur.

Yet, instead of the ladies turning all their attention to this, and organising a midwifery school of the highest efficiency in both science and practice, they enter men's classes, and lectures, and examinations, which don't wish to have them, and say they want the same education as men.

Then, is there not an immense confusion as to whether they are ever to be called in as medical attendants to men?

'No,' say those lady doctors who have at all thought out the question. 'We wish to be educated as if we were going to attend men, but we should think it an insult to be called in to attend men.'

Why not adjourn for a century, or for half a century, the question whether *all* branches of medical and surgical practice shall be exercised by women, even upon women? It is a question which may safely be left to settle itself.

But here is a matter so pressing, so universal, so universally recognised, viz., the preferable attendance of women upon women in midwifery, that it may really be summed up thus:—Although every woman would prefer a woman to attend upon her in her lying-in, and in diseases peculiar to her and her children, yet the woman does not exist, or hardly exists, to do it. Midwives are so ignorant that it is almost a term of contempt.

The rich woman cannot find fully qualified women, but only men to attend her, and the poor woman only takes unqualified women because she cannot afford to pay well-qualified men.

But why should the midwives be ignorant? and why (in the great movement that there is now to make women into medical men) should not this branch, midwifery, which they will find no one to contest against them—not at least in the estimation of the patients—be the first ambition of cultivated women? Is there any rational doubt that, suppose there were a man and a woman, both equally versed in midwifery art and science, the woman would be the one sent for by all lying-in women?

There is a better thing than making women into medical men, and that is making them into medical *women*.

Surely it is the first object to enable women, by the most thorough training, practical and scientific, to practise that branch of the art of medicine which all are agreed should be theirs, *not* ' like men ' —for nearly all the best men are agreed how deficient are the practical training and opportunities of medical students, especially in midwifery, which deficiency yet does not prevent them from obtaining diploma, license, all they want, in order to practise—*not* ' like men ' then, but like *women*, like women who wish to be real physician accoucheuses; that is, to attend and to be ' consulted in all deliveries, abnormal as well as normal, in diseases of women and children, as the best accoucheurs attend and are consulted.

Sensible women say, 'But the only means to obtain a scientific education *is* to enter men's classes.'

Is that the case?

Is the student's scientific and practical education all that could be wished?

Could there not be given (and *is* there not given, in some Continental schools?) a far more thorough and complete scientific education, as well as practical, where there are none but women, in a midwifery school, without all this struggle and contest, which raises questions so disagreeable and ridiculous that a woman of delicate feeling shuns the indelicacy of the contest—*not* the indelicacy of the occupation?

The parody, the *qui pro quo*, is a curious one.

The indelicacy of a man attending a woman in her lying-in is by necessity overlooked.

The indelicacy of a woman attending with men in medical classes is made much of.

Would it not be far better to get rid of both at once? to have women—trained with women, by women—to attend women—trained in all branches of a scientific and practical midwifery education?

But let no one think that real midwifery education can be less complete and thorough for a woman than it ought to be for a man, if women are really to be physician accoucheuses.

And let no one think that two or three courses of lectures—a month, three months, six months at a lying-in institution, con-ducting twenty, thirty, or one hundred labours—will make a woman into a (real) midwife.

One hundred labours may be normal, requiring no interference but that which a good midwifery nurse can give. The one hundred and first may be abnormal and may cost the patient her life or health, the attendant her reputation and peace, if her education has been nothing but the few lectures, the few weeks, the few labours.

Let us suppose for a moment that, leaving aside the ordinary talk of giving a woman a ' man's medical education,' good or bad, we imagine what a college might be to give the whole necessary training—medical, scientific and practical—to make real midwives, real physician accoucheuses.

There must be first, of course, the lying-in institution, the deliveries conducted by fully qualified head midwives, of whom enough perhaps exist already for this purpose, who will give practical instruction to the pupil midwives at the bedside.

There must be a staff of professors, to give scientific instruction in midwifery, but also in anatomy, physiology, and the like; in pathology and pathological branches; above all, in *sanitary* science and practice.

Dissections and post-mortem examinations will have to be practised. It need not be said that these must be at a quite different time and place in the ' course of education ' from the training about the lying-in patients.

Probably all these professors, or nearly all, must at first be men.

Probably in time all these professors, or nearly all, will come to be women.

The course of education, before the end of which no pupil can receive the certificate of a fully qualified midwife, must certainly not be less than two years.

Is this merely an ideal ?   *Is* it an Utopia?   Have we never seen it in practice ?   Could it not be put in practice in practical England ?

Seen it in practice we have—save and except the *sanitary* practice, which is wofully deficient—on the continent of Europe.

And lady professors there have been in midwifery on the Continent quite equal to the most distinguished physician accoucheurs in this or in any other country ; who took their place among these, among the Sir James Simpsons and the Sir Charles Lococks, as *of* them, and not outside of them, in all midwifery matters, scientific as well as practical.

The names of Madame Boivin and Madame Lachapelle, of Paris, are known to all Europe. And there are many other names of lady professors in midwifery and of midwives, not known in England at all, who take their uncontested places on the continent in practice, in consultation, in teaching, as a Sir James Simpson here. They teach in midwives' colleges, and imperial and royal ladies *are* sometimes, and often wish to be always, attended by them.

Note.—A society has already existed for several years, the object of which, according to its programme, is ' to provide educated women with proper facilities for learning the theory and practice of midwifery, and the accessory branches of medical science.'

The programme states most justly that, for want of these, for want of ' proper means of study,' of ' any public examination,' ' any person may undertake the duties of a midwife.'

Let us look what the ' proper means of study ' are which it provides.

They are—1. Attendance upon lectures during two winter sessions. 2. Attendance ' during the intervening summer' upon clinical practice at ' *a* ' lying-in hospital or maternity charity, with personal attendance upon at least *twenty-five* deliveries !

[It is easy to make a rough calculation how many cases of abnormal parturition occur to how many normal. Is it likely that among ' twenty-five deliveries ' there will be abnormal cases enough to practise the pupil-judgment, the pupil-hand ?]

These ladies have not even the advantages which the idlest student can hardly help availing himself of—and *his* minimum is ' three years.' Yet this is the course proposed to enable a woman to ' practise midwifery,' even in the sense in which we understand a man to ' practise midwifery,'—to enable a woman to become a

physician accoucheuse (for these ladies are expressly styled 'accoucheuses') in the sense in which we understand a man to be a
physician accoucheur.

The paper states, doubtless with truth, that these ladies 'are
the best taught accoucheuses hitherto accessible to the English
public.' May we not hope that, in future years, the society will
be enabled to give 'accoucheuses' still better taught 'to the
English public'?

LONDON : PRINTED BY
SPOTTISWOODE AND CO., NEW-STREET SQUARE
AND PARLIAMENT STREET

Printed in the United States
By Bookmasters